BROKEN AND BRAVE

THE FIGHT TO HEAL AMERICAN HEALTHCARE

TIFFANY L SMITH, RN

BROKEN AND BRAVE HEALTH, LLC

Copyright © 2025 by Tiffany L Smith, RN

All rights reserved.

No part of this book may be reproduced in any form or by any electronic or mechanical means, including information storage and retrieval systems, without written permission from the author, except for the use of brief quotations in a book review.

For every provider who's been asked, "What could you have done better?"
For every patient labeled non-compliant.
For the families told to "trust the process" as it destroyed someone they loved.
And for every soul who dared to question the system—this book is for you.
You are not broken.
You are brave.

CONTENTS

Acknowledgments	vii
Preface	ix

PART I
A Day in the Life of a COVID Nurse — 1

PART TWO
THE RUDDERLESS SHIP

1. Fear and Resilience	91
2. Burnout	117
3. Behind the Scrubs	127
4. Nurses' Proverbial Plates	141
5. The Cost of Care	157
6. The Overworked, Underpaid, and Indispensable CNAs	167
7. From Healers to Hustlers	173
8. Partnering for Progress	185
9. Predatory Power	193
10. A System That Pretends to Care	205
11. Health as Rebellion	223
12. A Broken System and a Nation in Crisis	233
Notes	261

ACKNOWLEDGMENTS

To the nurses I've worked alongside:

You cracked jokes in the chaos, covered me when I couldn't keep going, and reminded me I wasn't alone. You changed my life, and I will never forget you. Thank you.

To my kids:

Thank you for walking through the fire with me and emerging stronger, kinder, and more incredible than I could have imagined. You are my reason, my heart, and my revolution. I love you.

To my husband:

Your support has been unwavering, your belief in me unshakable. It is an honor to be loved by you, and to love you in return.

To my mom:

You've always had patience as I moved through each stage of life, always picked up the phone, and gave my emotions a safe place to land. Your faith in me—and your trust that I can handle anything—created the foundation for this book. I can't thank you enough. I love you.

To my dad:

Our fire seems to burn at the same intensity. You always offer sound advice and have always believed I could do anything a man can do. Thank you for that. I love you.

To my brother:

You created the cover that holds this fire. I'm so proud we

did this together. I love knowing you're always there, even though we live far apart. I'm proud of the man and dad you've become. Thank you. I love you.

To my editors:

Marieke, thank you for sticking with the project, even when it didn't feel up your alley at first. You helped shape this book into what it became.

Paul, thank you for your creative touch, digital expertise, and for helping make my blabbering more succinct. This book is so much better after being in your hands.

PREFACE

When I first thought about writing this book, I had no idea where to begin. I wasn't looking to write a tell-all complaint-fest about being a nurse (though I have plenty I could say), and I wasn't trying to stir up controversy just for the sake of it. I certainly wasn't aiming to jeopardize my job or paint a target on my back. But I couldn't ignore the pull any longer—this internal push to speak the truth. So, I started writing. Hesitantly at first, but with growing clarity and conviction, because silence wasn't an option anymore.

In healthcare, questioning the system can feel dangerous. Being labeled "medically dissident" isn't just a buzzword—it's a threat. Those of us who dare to challenge the status quo are often dismissed, silenced, or punished. The truth is, medicine in the US isn't just flawed—it's rigged.

Government agencies, research institutions, pharmaceutical companies, and media conglomerates are all tangled up in a web of profit and power. What gets studied, published, or shared with the public is carefully curated. Research is funded based on the likelihood that it will produce the "right" answer for the funder. Results are buried, cherry-picked, or massaged to look a certain way. Even our search engines feed us filtered information. And medical journals? Once pillars of objectivity—now often puppets of corporate sponsorship.

As a nurse with a deep commitment to humanity, I struggle to accept that this is the system we're expected to trust. I understand the motives—power, money, control—but I can't reconcile them with the human cost. Why do we allow this? Why is critical thinking discouraged in a field that should thrive on curiosity and integrity? Why are dissenting voices—often those advocating for patients, equity, or reform—the ones most aggressively silenced?

That's why this book exists. It's a call to think, to question, and to feel. To pull back the curtain on the messy, broken and beautiful chaos of healthcare and ask:

What the hell are we doing—and why aren't we fixing it?

The book is split into two parts. The first is a raw, unfiltered narrative of a single twelve-hour shift as a nurse in the middle of the COVID-19 pandemic. It's timestamped, real-time, and brutally honest. You'll walk with me through the rooms, the heartbreak, the bodily fluids, the codes, the brief moments of joy, and the silent grief that follows me home. It's a snapshot of a world most people never see—but desperately need to.

The second part zooms out to explore the broader dysfunction that fuels the chaos we experience on the frontlines. I examine everything from the insurance industry's chokehold on care to the predatory practices of pharmaceutical companies, to the dangerous silence surrounding healthcare worker abuse, burnout, and moral injury. This part of the book is research-driven, solution-focused, and unapologetically bold in calling out the rot at the core of the system.

My hope is that this book does more than just inform. I want it to awaken.

To empower nurses and doctors to speak up.

To encourage patients to ask better questions.

To inspire anyone with a pulse to stop sleepwalking through a system that profits from our suffering and demand something better—for ourselves and each other.

If you're a healthcare worker, I hope this book helps you feel seen, validated, and strengthened. If you're a patient—or just a person trying to live a healthy life in this country—I hope this gives you tools to protect yourself, advocate for better care, and take control of your health before the system takes control of you.

And if you're pissed off by the time you finish reading it?

Good. That means you're awake. That means we're getting somewhere.

If any part of this book speaks to you—if you have a story to share, a question to ask, or a desire to take back your health and start a new path—I'd love to hear from you. You can reach me at brokenandbravehealth@gmail.com. Whether it's to share your experience, begin a conversation, or explore holistic ways to get off medications, improve your overall physical health, improve your mental health, and regain control—I'm here for that.

We all deserve better. Let's start with the truth.

Tiffany Smith
May 2025

PART ONE

A DAY IN THE LIFE OF A COVID NURSE

NOVEMBER 28, 2020

5:25 AM

Alarm. I press snooze.

Ugh. Okay, let's set the tone. I will be positive and set myself up for success.

I am a nurse and have been for over a decade. I work in a hospital on the medical-surgical floor, and today I am starting my fourth twelve-hour shift in a row.

I roll over and sit on the side of my bed for a minute in the darkness like a gremlin. I rub the sleep out of my eyes and see my sweet dog Bella raising her head and looking at me like, "not again, wtf."

I sit on my bed for a few more seconds and then lay my head down on my pillow again, being sure to keep my legs out of the covers so I don't fall back to sleep.

Man, am I exhausted.

My alarm goes off again, and I curse at it as I turn it off and actually stand up this time.

I rub more sleep out of my eyes and yawn as I shuffle into the bathroom and turn on the disgustingly bright light.

Who on planet earth decided that seven-seven shifts were the way to go for healthcare? Who was like, "YES! Get to work in the dark and leave work in the dark for most of the year! It's so fun!"

I would like to punch them in the tit.

I stand there in the bathroom and let my eyes adjust to the brightness. I look in the mirror and shake my head. I mean, truly, I am a sight to behold at 5:35 am.

I brush my teeth and then go into the kitchen to start a cup of coffee. I yawn again, and Bella stares at me as if she's never eaten a day in her life.

I make her sit while I get her food ready and then release her to eat. I stand there listening to her crunch down her breakfast, and then suddenly remember I have an actual job and responsibilities and have to leave in like 20 minutes.

I quickly make my cup of coffee and go back into the bathroom, put moisturizer on my dry face, and do a very quick, very basic makeup job.

My entire "beauty routine" takes about eight minutes. This includes a tiny bit of concealer on my red spots, a touch of blush so I can pretend to be mostly alive, a tad of light eye shadow in a sad attempt to brighten my eyes, and a single layer of mascara. I put my hair back into a low secure bun because I will have to put it into my COVID scrub cap for my entire shift, so it doesn't matter what it looks like.

I get dressed in my lovely scrubs that I am so sick of wearing. I don't really know how to dress when I'm not in scrubs. I feel pretty proud if I manage to put together an entire outfit that doesn't include a sweatshirt or leggings of some kind.

I look at my collection of bright, neon-colored sneakers that I am famous for at work and decide on the lime-green ones today. I always try to make my secondary mask (the one over my N95) match my sneakers. Lots of people on my floor look forward to it and comment on it. They are also sure to comment when they do not match, just to make sure I know that I'm slacking.

I get a kick out of it, and I love wearing bright things, so, meh, why not?

I stand in front of my full-length mirror. In scrubs. Coffee in hand. Exhaustion on my face. What a familiar sight.

I suddenly remember deodorant, which I am eternally grateful for, and apply some. I stare into my eyes in the bathroom mirror and see the absorbed suffering deep inside of them.

The things I have seen as a nurse—taking on the trauma, pain, confusion, and overall grief—has taken a huge toll on my soul. I know that I am meant to do this; I am a damn good nurse. But, shit, there has to be a limit to what we are expected to endure, right?

I am even pretty good at self-care. I try to be outside whenever I can. I try to surround myself with beauty and happiness in all the aspects of my life. But it's never enough to shake the knowledge that soon I will be back under the glare of the hospital's fluorescent lights, absorbing and enduring and performing once again.

I nod at myself in the mirror and then go make more coffee—my 32-ouncer for the ride into work and the beginning of my day. Once procured, I get into my car and let it idle for a sec to warm it up. It's a chilly morning. I rub my hands together and then stick them under my thighs.

Pulling out of the driveway, I mourn the fact that I am not snuggled in my bed.

On my way, I am already going through the steps of the day, mentally preparing for the likely fuckery that will ensue the moment I walk onto the floor. My brain is still full from my last shift, and I will probably have the same assignment as yesterday, so I start to put my to-do list together in my head. At that point, I realize that I can't remember anything because my brain is always foggy, exhausted, and overwhelmed. So, I eagerly grab my phone and use the voice-to-text in my Notes app and verbalize my plan and hopes for the day.

LOL. Just kidding. I rock out to some early 2000s grunge music while chugging my coffee like it's the last cup I will ever have and doing my best to not think about the shitshow I'm about to walk into.

I park in the employee parking garage and walk quickly towards the hospital, hoping not to get assaulted by a hidden thug.

Shit. I realize as I see the door that I forgot my ID—can't get in without that.

I go back to my car and grab my ID badge, looking around as if something else will magically pop out of the abyss of my vehicle, saying, "You forgot me too!" Nothing does, so I start speed-walking again and say a little prayer to the nursing gods to please allow me to have a smooth shift.

Fourth shift in a row. *I just need a smooth day. Please: God, universe, whoever; please.*

I swear, if Tim pisses in his water cup ONE MORE TIME, I will just lose my shit. Like, utterly lose it.

It is freaking cold today, so I hustle even faster to the employee entrance, scan my badge, and enter. It smells like cardboard boxes and sanitizer. *Ahh, the scent of mental instability and depression.*

I take the stairs to my floor because I am trying to be fit. My feet already hurt, and I've been standing for like five minutes. I get to the floor and instantly hear the dinging of a call light.

It's fine. I love this sound. I don't have nightmares and dreams literally centered around this sound AT ALL. It is the sound of my people. Honestly, I can't even hear it after a while on the floor, but right at this moment, it makes me want to ninja-kick someone in the throat.

As I'm walking to the break room, a CNA (certified nursing assistant) speeds by me, trying to answer one of the three call lights. She hits me on the arm, "Welcome to the shitshow."

Word. I knew it.

I get to the break room and look at my watch. It's 6:35 am. I can't punch-in until 6:38 because, you know, HR. I put my stuff in my locker, get my pens, scissors, penlight, doctor's stethoscope, ChapStick, and random IV saline flushes I had from yesterday, and shove them in my scrub pockets. Found a bonus stack of wrinkly alcohol pads too, so I put those in my little front pocket that is otherwise useless.

I get my N95 mask that I have used for the past three twelve-hour shifts and put it on. It smells like coffee and diarrhea. I take it off and put some peppermint essential oil in it that my mom sent me and then remember to put my foam pad over my nose to protect it from getting rubbed raw from the mask. I put the mask back on, clamp it down tight so there are no air leaks, put my lime-green medical mask over it, and look in my mini locker mirror.

Sexy.

6:38 am. Okay. I scan my badge, punch in, and take a deep breath with my eyes closed. As I am trying to savor my Zen breath, I inhale the smell of a fresh shit a patient must have just taken. Or an ostomy bag being emptied—impossible to tell.

Our new grad nurse comes into the break room. I call her

"our" because she is our little baby nurse. Look at her. Perfect messy bun that is literally not messy. Are her scrubs ironed?? Oh, and those brand-new Dansko clogs. She even has an engraved stethoscope label with her name and "RN" on it. I bet her mom had it made for her when she graduated. Or grandma.

Part of me is jealous; her makeup-laden fresh, bright eyes. But another, larger part of me knows that she will look like me in just a couple of short years. Or a couple of short months.

I look in the tiny mirror again, and I see a messy bun that is actually messy, bags beneath the used-to-be-bright blue eyes; all with a beautiful undertone of mental exhaustion, no fucks given, and loathing that only a seasoned nurse can achieve.

I open the break room door and step onto the unit.

I work on the medical-surgical floor of a Level I trauma center. We are currently smack-bang in the middle of our "COVID surge" and, folks, it is *no bueno*.

My unit has become the COVID med-surg unit, and let me tell you, it's a real treat. I have been here for five years. I used to really love it here, but the burnout is real. COVID-19 has been a life- and career-changer for nurses across the globe, and my floor is no exception. We are all deadass tired, for real. We have all had enough. We are so fucking sick of watching people die, of watching people go from walking and talking to intubated and dead. I've been a nurse for twelve years, but I have thought multiple times about going back to waitressing. Or starting an OnlyFans account, I'm not sure yet.

I head to the nurses' station and try to find my assignment, but the charge nurse is still working on it because three people died overnight. Juggling rooms, their cleaning, and who gets the next available bed is a completely shit job. I am so thankful I am not her.

I hear a chair alarm go off and walk up to the door of the room to find an elderly patient trying to get up on their own.

Jesus, Mildred, I know you have to pee but dang, hang on a hot second. I open the door a tiny crack and yell, "Wait for me, Mildred!"

Thankfully, she sits back down.

I put on all my PPE (Personal Protective Equipment) and go in. I help her to the bathroom and wait patiently as she tries to do it on her own. 'Cause you know, independence. I end up having to help her anyhow, 'cause, you know, weakness.

Approximately seventy-three hours later, I walk her back to her chair and make sure she's comfortable. I get her blanket from the CNA who brought it to me, put her feet up, place her table back over her lap, and make sure her nurse call button, phone, and menu are all in reach. She wants to order breakfast ASAP because she is STARVINGGGG. She reminds me of my sweet dog Bella, acting as if she has never eaten before a day in her life.

She also demands an additional warm blanket because, she says, "this place is an ice box unless you're fat."

I press the call button and ask someone to bring me a warm blanket because I'm already gowned-up in here.

She informs me that her nurse yesterday was "very bitchy and pushy."

I ask her to tell me more, and she says that the nurse made her get up and move around and kept coming in to bother her and make her do things she didn't want to do. I empathize with Mildred, saying it does sound like her nurse yesterday was in fact a bitch.

It was me. I was yesterday's nurse.

6:55 AM

My assignment is ready. Seven patients. Jesus. Day #4, and seven patients to take care of.

It's fine. I had six yesterday, and only had to drink an entire bottle of wine last night to wash away all the thoughts of shit I missed or didn't do perfectly throughout the day, so what's one more?

Maybe tonight will be vodka and a crappy movie.

I find the night nurse I need to get report from. *Because of COVID, we do walking reports from the doorways.

I am diligent about keeping each patient's whiteboard up-to-date for fear of administrative wrath. *What's the date?* Every day runs together lately.

Whiteboards are the bane of my existence. There is SO MUCH information on them, and the patients and family members don't even read them, they just ask me.

Like, yeah . . . let me take the time to write every single detail of what's going on with your body on this board for it to be ignored, that's cool.

My nighttime counterpart hands me the work phone as I scan my report sheets. I have seven COVID-positive patients. All of them have multiple comorbidities on top of their COVID. This means that they have multiple serious diagnoses that greatly affect their prognosis. I know all of them except Ron in room 113.

My report sheet looks like this:

1. **Mildred:** Room 106. COVID, septic, wound on foot. *need surgical consult*
2. **Roxy:** Room 112. COVID, new-onset diabetic/kidney failure. *blood sugars brittle and unstable*

---

* *Get report*: when the off-going nurse tells the oncoming nurse what's going on with their patients.

3. **Jerry:** Room 110. COVID, bariatric/diverticulitis. *surgery today*
4. **Ron:** Room 113. COVID, severe diarrhea. *dehydration*
5. **Barbara:** Room 111. COVID, end-stage lung cancer. *family meeting today*
6. **Tim:** Room 114. COVID, continuous BiPAP.
7. **Juan:** Room 109. COVID, severe dementia. *minimal oxygen*

All of them are sick. So sick. But the entire floor—hell, the entire hospital—is full of super-sick people, so it is what it is.

More often than not, we used to get patients who had just one thing wrong with them. But Americans are so incredibly unhealthy now that this is rare, and our hospital is always full of acutely ill people.

I try to get a more detailed report at the nurses' station, but it's a total shitshow because I am following one of those nurses who is a hot-ass mess even when she's really trying *not* to be. Her papers are disorganized and have unidentifiable stains on them. She keeps getting patients mixed up while talking, and she is so exhausted and mentally drained that she just desperately wants to go home.

Right now, she can't stop talking about the fact that Tim keeps pissing in his water cup, and I'm like, "I KNOW RIGHT?? How can a fully alert and oriented man just keep pissing where he is supposed to be drinking from?"

She says that last night she got him a fresh cup and TWO urinals—one for each side of his bed—filled his cup up with water for him to DRINK and an hour later, he opened his cup and pissed in it, ON TOP OF the water already in there, causing everything to overflow all over his bed.

Bro. I can't even. . . .

She finishes, giving me a half-assed report on the rest of my people and apologizes for being a mess. I automatically forgive her because, girl, we all are.

Hot Mess goes into the corner to finish her documentation, and I open the electronic medical record and scan through my patients' medications on my handheld. As I'm doing this, a call bell goes off.

It's another nurse who needs help with a patient. I poke my head in the cubicle curtain, "What's up?"

Stacy—a brilliantly smart, witty 35-year-old woman—looks up at me from the patient's bedside and says, "I need towels, soap, Chux, a new gown, and all new bedding. There's been an explosion."

Perfect. I go to the supply closet, shaking my head at the massive amounts of diarrhea that COVID seems to give people. Like, if there were a world record for shitting the bed, Ron in 113 would most definitely hold it.

I get all the supplies from the supply closet and start the donning process. I put on my shoe protectors and sanitize my hands. I already have a surgical cap on, so I go right to my garbage-bag gown. (They aren't actually made of garbage bags, but that is exactly what they feel like.)

I feel like a garbage princess every time I tie myself up in one of these bitches. Putting on a pair of gloves, I hook my thumb into the garbage bag thumb hole, then put on eye protection, then my second pair of gloves. I adjust my N95 so I'm sure there are no leaks, grab my armful of supplies, and head in.

We clean the patient up while both working up a hell of a sweat. We finally get him all clean and fresh, but that dreaded smell still permeates the air.

We look around and . . . *urghhhhh.* More shit.

Stacy and I have both been nurses for years, so we are not new to this kind of fuckery. It becomes second nature to just assume that nothing will ever go to plan, so you become much more chill and (let's face it) less uptight when things like this happen. We call for more supplies and start the process over again.

We banter while changing him again and it strikes me how we hardly need to speak to coordinate what we are doing, it has become second nature.

She tells me she is thinking of taking a traveling contract so that she can work a few hours away from home and make more than double her wage here.

I mean, why wouldn't you?

As I am wiping ass, I think, *why, oh why did I go to school for this?*

School was false advertising, yo. I was told CNAs mostly do this, but we have been so understaffed with CNAs that they basically don't exist anymore. I mean, I wouldn't do that job for as little as they get paid knowing McDonalds is offering $1,000 sign-on bonuses and $20 an hour. Hmm . . . clean people's asses and get bitched at all day long for $16 an hour or flip burgers and risk possibly getting acne because of grease for $20 an hour?

Easy decision. Can't blame them but, damn, it never ends.

Finally, we are done. I look at Stacy and say, "I'm out. Been a pleasure doing business with you." I rip off my gown and gloves, put them in the overflowing trash can, and leave.

Why is the trash always full? Oh, that's right—we also have almost no environmental service (EVS) technicians to clean our rooms, for the same reason we have so few CNAs.

Word.

I go into the medication (med) room, walk over to the locked medication machine (called a "Pyxis") and start getting medications for my first patient. As I'm doing this, my work phone rings. It's room 110.

My bariatric patient, Jerry, wants his pain pill. NOW. I look in his medication record, and he literally just got one from night shift less than an hour ago. I stop what I'm doing and get his morning pills together, gown up, and go into his room to explain what the deal is with this pain pill schedule. Just like I did 47 times yesterday. He hasn't stopped ringing his call light for the pill, and the floor secretary is starting to lose her mind.

He accuses me of lying and says he did not get a pill one hour ago, and the other nurse must be a liar too. He starts yelling and carrying on, and telling me this hospital isn't shit, and he hates it, and we never do what he wants or needs. Tells me that I have no idea what I'm doing and must not be able to read.

Well, fuck me, then. It's like, dude, then leave! Please do me the favor of getting out of here so we can all take better care of people who appreciate us and want our help. This is not a hotel; I do not provide room service, nor am I a drug dealer that you call up when you are jonesing. I am a medical professional, and you should be required to treat me as such.

Instead of saying this, I just say, "Okay, Jerry. I'll let the doc know you'd like to change the frequency of your pills, just like I did yesterday. He said you are maxed-out on your narcotics last time I asked, and he said he will not be increasing your dose—but today is a new day!"

Between being called a smartass and a bitch, I ask him what his pain level is. He tells me it is ten-out-of-ten—i.e., the worst pain he has ever felt in his life—as he plays Mahjong on his phone and sips on a nice cold Coke someone must have brought him. With ice.

I wish someone would bring me a nice cold beverage. With vodka.

I lower my eyelids and have no fucks left in my voice when

I say, "Jerry, you're telling me that your pain is so severe that you feel as if you're being cut open with a chainsaw right now?"

And he lets me know that YES, it is, and if I wasn't such an incompetent idiot, I wouldn't have to ask him that question.

Cool.

Grabbing my stethoscope off my neck, I do my initial head-to-toe morning assessment on him and attempt to listen to his lungs and heart and abdomen for bowel sounds. Unfortunately, when someone is as large as this guy is, it's much more difficult to hear these organs. The amount of space between the stethoscope and the organ is so vast that it's really hard to pick up on what could be potentially life-saving, subtle changes.

Needless to say, I get degraded throughout the entire assessment and don't find anything new on examination.

Sitting the mini cup in front of him, I ask him to take his morning medication that I pulled for him. After another three minutes or so of him telling me how stupid I am, and how shitty this hospital is, he finally takes them.

Why THANK YOU SIR for being so kind and easy to deal with. It is patients like this that make me want to put my middle finger up and walk out, only to never come back ever again.

Taking off my garbage outfit, I walk out of his room and try to figure out what to do next.

As I'm turning around to walk back to the med room, the one and only CNA on the floor for the day—Dee—comes running up to me to tell me that room 112's blood pressure (BP) is a very low 82/58, and yes, she's sure because she checked it in both arms twice.

Crap. The nursing gods must have had their headphones in earlier when I was talking to them, *what the hell?*

We go into the room together after gowning up, and I assess my sweet 42-year-old female patient, Roxy. She's drowsy and slurring her speech and is disoriented. I tell the CNA to get the glucometer and then check her sugar level: 39.*

Awesome. This is low, way too low. I degown, go get some orange juice and glucagon (artificial sugar), get gowned back up, head back into her room, and have her take them both as quickly as possible. I encourage fluids because I'm assuming she is also dehydrated with such a low BP.

Dee goes to get some fresh water for me, and I put the straw up to her lips. Roxy looks up at me with doe eyes, and I can tell she is scared. I quietly reassure her that I've got her, and I won't let anything happen to her. Within minutes she starts to calm down, and I hear a call for help down the hall. I ask Dee to stay with the patient and recheck her blood sugar level in ten minutes.

"If you need anything, call me, but don't leave her side."

I know this leaves the rest of the floor short on CNA coverage, but I need someone with Roxy—she's a newly diagnosed diabetic, and seems to have brittle blood sugars because this is the fifth time in four days that I've had to give her artificial sugar.

I text the doc as I'm walking to the next patient's room about the BP and glucose level. I ask if he wants a bolus of IV fluids to see if we can pull her BP up a little. He responds with a "yes, give her a bolus" and a thumbs-up about her glucose level and the interventions I've already done.

Looking up and down the hall, I try to find where the call for help came from and see people running to a room. I follow them and quickly look through the small window on the door, and New Grad is standing over her patient, who looks to be unresponsive. I am the third RN there, and we are all gowning and gloving as quickly as possible. The first RN gets in the

---

* mg/dL (*milligrams per deciliter*)

room, checks for a pulse and—not finding one—presses the "code blue" button.

The team is activated, and I grab the code cart and step into the room with another coworker. Over the next several minutes, the patient is worked; CPR (cardiopulmonary resuscitation), drugs, more IVs are started, and doctors (fellows and residents) gather trying to be a part of the excitement.

LOL, excitement. That should *not* be a word used when someone is dead.

Did you know that someone who needs CPR is dead? Not dying, but *dead*. We are literally trying to bring them back from the dead.

Multiple emergency carts are pushed in and crowd the room. *Why are the wheels on these things always so loud?* All kinds of equipment wrappers, saline flushes, syringes, and garbage is being thrown all over the floor, the bed, and the tables as supplies are unwrapped and equipment is hooked up. He is stripped naked and his privates are just out and flopping around. None of us even bat an eye.

A phlebotomist is attempting to draw blood from a vein while the patient's chest is being compressed and he is bouncing all over the place. People are trying to remain calm, while running a code all dressed like trash bags.

We are all sweating profusely.

I am the drug pusher, so I listen to instructions from the lead doc and push lifesaving medications whenever called for.[*] New Grad is in the corner with her beautiful eyes all wide and terrified. This is her first code. It will not be her last. I try to give her a small, crooked smile that says, "It'll be okay, just hang

---

[*] *Push*: the rapid injection of a drug directly into the bloodstream, usually through an intravenous (IV) line.

in there," but I can't because of this damned mask. *COVID is so awesome.*

Anne, the floor secretary, is doing compressions and is rotating with a male travel nurse whose name I don't remember. The CPR feedback monitor keeps saying, "Good compressions," as if it's some weird emotional support dog that can speak.

After a 20-minute-plus attempt at resuscitating the patient, we fail. Time of death is called.

I am sweating so badly because of this garbage bag dress that it's dripping down my back. I start peeling off my protective layers and notice that the medium gloves box is empty. I go to the clean utility room, grab a new box, and replace it.

As the famous meme says, I am the backbone of this hospital.

I am reeling and feel lost and confused standing in the hallway with no direct purpose for a second. *Where was I? What was I doing?*

It's so bizarre to be part of a traumatic death like that and then step into the hallway back to complete normalcy. As if I didn't just push enough epinephrine to restart six horses' hearts. As if we didn't just crack every piece of cartilage and probably some bones in that man's chest. As if I didn't just watch his naked body get flopped around and pushed down on while being poked and prodded and shocked and broken. As if I didn't have to regulate my own nervous system over and over while also remembering algorithms and proper procedures and then performing them correctly.

As if someone hadn't just died.

Oh—Roxy!

I jog back to room 112 to check on her. I start to gown and glove, but it takes me a while because my hands are so sweaty from the code. Thinking maybe the alcohol will dry them out, I put another layer of sanitizer on my hands. It works well enough for me to get my gloves on.

Walking in the room, I see she is up and talking again and is stable. Dee reports a sugar of 78 when she checked it again. I thank her sincerely. I tell her she is good to go to her other patients because I know her workload is completely out of hand if mine is this ridiculous.

Rechecking Roxy's sugar, I see it's 102. Crisis averted, for now. While I'm in there, I do my morning assessment on her as well. While her heart rate is a little slow, nothing sounds obviously abnormal to me. Her blood pressure after all this drama is 98/71, which is much more acceptable.

My phone vibrates in my pocket. It's a message from lab—they tell me the blood samples drawn by the night shift from my patient in room 111's PICC line were "hemolyzed" and need to be redrawn. *What the HELL does hemolyzed mean?* I should look it up, but I swear it's like the lab loves to play games. I bet they say the same shit about us, though. *This is ridic.* As I am typing my very polite answer that I will redraw it gladly, the phone rings.

The unit secretary says Juan in room 109 wants to know where his wife is and if anyone is going to come to see him today. I start towards the med room, but when I get there, I have to wait for another nurse to finish up before I can take all of Juan's meds out of the Pyxis.

Walking to the room, I get gowned up again and enter.

Juan starts telling me everything about his children and family and how he wishes they would come and visit him. He has pretty late-stage dementia. I want to explain to him that he has COVID, and that visitors aren't allowed. Instead, I tell him that his wife is coming later today but is busy at the moment.

When people have dementia, it is much better to live in their reality than attempt to bring them into yours.

He gets teary and his eyes drop to the floor, and he says, "Why is she not here right now?" Sighing, I sit down next to him, and rub his back gently as he takes his pills. The rustling from my garbage bag is really soothing, I'm sure. I'm also sure that me being covered literally head to toe in this equipment is disorienting as hell for someone that is already disoriented to begin with.

I tell him calmly that everything will be okay, and that his family will be here soon. He nods slowly and closes his eyes. Even though nursing has made me jaded and pissed off at the world, it is moments like this that I cherish. It feels like I make at least a tiny bit of a difference.

I take off my gear and back out of the door while turning down the lights. When I turn around, New Grad is standing right behind me and scares the shit out of me. *Jesus!* I see a limp smile in her eyes behind her mask, but she is crying and asks for help because she has never had to speak to a family with this kind of news before.

She says, "The doctor already talked to the wife, but now she and the daughter want to talk to me because I've been his nurse for the last three days. We built such a great rapport over the phone trying to get him better, I don't think I can face them alone."

I tell her we will do it together, and we head to a secluded spot behind the nurses' station and pick up the phone. She needs to get used to doing this on her own, but I wish that someone had sat with me the first time I had to do it, so I sacrifice my precious time for our baby nurse.

The family is devastated, obviously. They are looking for any kind of comfort they can get in this shitty situation that no one can control. They want to hear that we did everything, and that no, they aren't bad people because they weren't by his side. They crave a nurse's steadfastness, calm, and knowledge in their time of crisis. They rely on us to be a pillar of strength and speak to them in terms that they can understand.

They ask New Grad more questions, and she starts to cry with them. The patient's wife of 50 years is sobbing and quietly says, "I just wish I could have seen him one last time before he died."

I know. I am so sorry. No visitors because of COVID, so your husband of FIFTY YEARS died without you in a strange hospital bed surrounded by walking garbage bags, and you didn't get to say goodbye.

So. Fucking. Awful.

Eventually, we give our respects and well wishes to the rest of the family and hang up. I give New Grad a hug, tell her it will be okay, and that she needs to suck it up and move on to take care of her other patients.

We wipe our tears, fix our masks, and try to re-orient ourselves again.

As if someone hadn't just died.

8:30 AM

Lord Almighty, it's only 8:30. How can so many things happen in such a short amount of time?

My stomach is so empty that the acid from my enormous coffee is eating away at the lining. I wonder if an ulcer would qualify as workers' comp? Or at LEAST get me some paid time off?

Okay, so I have so far only given meds to two out of seven patients. Time to fix that—they are due by 9:00 am.

I go to the Pyxis and pull out Roxy's medications. I make sure to grab the bag of IV fluid called "lactated ringers" (LR fluid) for the bolus the doc ordered earlier. Gowning up and going into her room, I check her sugar again because she is technically due for insulin, which I am totally not comfortable giving her, after this morning's episode. (Insulin causes sugar to be sucked up by cells, reducing its level in the blood.) Her sugar is only 108, though, which means it's too low according to the sliding scale guidelines to give insulin, so I am in the clear.

    I scan all the meds and push them out of their packages into a tiny cup. When I give her the pills, she puts her hand on my arm and looks me in the eye. She whispers, "Thank you," and takes the meds. I know she is thanking me for more than just her pills, and squeeze her shoulder in response and turn to spike the IV bag with new tubing, prime it, and put it in the pump.

    Next, I clean her IV off with an alcohol wipe, then flush it, hook up the tubing, and press play on the pump. I triple-check the tubing, the pump, and the patient. I nod my head as she says thank you once again and quietly leave her room after making sure she has everything she needs, and that her call bell is in reach.

    I walk by the nurses' station to go back to the med room, and the unit secretary stops me and says that Theresa—the daughter of Mildred, my patient in room 106—is on the phone and has some concerns. My eyes roll alllll the way into the back of my head and I say, "Of course she does," because she does this shit every single day.

    Theresa is a nurse practitioner, so obviously she knows everything about medicine and nursing and believes that none of us know what we are doing, and that her mother is getting subpar care, and she would DEFINITELY be doing better if she was us.

    Isn't it interesting, though, that this lady will not actually care for her mom? Like . . . Mildred lives in a nursing home, not with her daughter. Mildred is pretty high functioning, but

Theresa placed her in a home because she was "too high-maintenance to manage at home." And yet, we are not good enough?

I have so many questions.

Mildred is here because she received a pressure injury to her heel and this led to a bacterial infection spreading in her blood (sepsis). She got COVID because it's impossible NOT to have COVID when you live in a nursing home nowadays.

How did she get septic even though she has 24-hour care at the nursing home, you ask? Well, brilliant Ms. Theresa kept telling the nursing home doctors that if SHE were providing care for her mother, SHE would be giving her a high dose of broad-spectrum antibiotics and keeping her out of the hospital at all costs because of COVID, and demanded that this is what they do.

Well, the doctor listened to her for a few days too long, and Mildred is now very sick here in paradise with me. I pick up the phone and get a lovely earful from Theresa about how her mother's blinds aren't even up yet, and it's past 8:30.

I tell her that it's been a crazy morning, and I haven't had a chance to get to her mom's morning routine yet. She tells me that when she was a floor nurse, she used to check on all her patients before starting any of her duties. I ask her if that was during a global pandemic and she reluctantly says no. I tell her we are taking very good care of her mom, and that I understand how stressful and scary it must be to not be able to see her in person. I tell her that I will go to Mildred's room next and ensure that her blinds are up to let in some light.

Theresa tries to make a list of all the things she wants me to do for her mom, but I interrupt her. I say, "I have multiple patients who all also need my attention. I will certainly take great care of your mom, and if anything comes up, I will call you."

She says okay and hangs up on me.

Word.

I get all Mildred's meds, gown up, and go into her room. Walking over to her window and opening the curtains, I ask her how she is feeling this morning. "Tired," she says.

Aren't we all?

She already has her antibiotic, vancomycin, running in her IV, so I check on that and make a mental note of about what time it will run out.

I do my morning head-to-toe assessment and don't find anything concerning and give her her pills, which is the ungodly amount of twelve, and she takes them. One. At. A. Time. If there were words for how excruciating a process this is, I would use them. It's like dying 1,000 deaths. It's like nails on a chalkboard. It's like peeling off your own fingernails.

Nope—none of these do it justice.

Also, why are nail injuries so yucky? I have seen some major shit in my career, but anything to do with a fingernail or toenail and I'm out. It makes me quiver because DAMN that's gotta hurt. Oh, also eyes. Eye traumas make me squirm majorly.

While standing there waiting on her, I look at her foot wound, and yes, it is indeed nasty and infected. It looks like her heel is actually rotting off. And smells like it too. Checking my handheld, I confirm that general surgery has been consulted, which they have, so we are just waiting on their assessment.

I wonder silently if Theresa will file a complaint later because of the blinds, but honestly who gives any shits about that at this point? After 525,600 minutes, Mildred is finally done with her pills. *Thank you, Jesus.*

As soon as I get into the hallway, New Grad tells me that Tim has pissed in his water cup again and now it's all over him, the bed, and the floor.

This is the day. This is when I go insane. Hook me up to an

IV sedation drip, slap me with a psychosis diagnosis, and bring me to the psych ward because I am LOSING MY MIND.

I go to the clean utility room and grab all new bedding and supplies, including towels to clean the floor with, and put them near room 114's door. Quickly grabbing his couple of pills, I go to gown and glove, and head into the room with this armful of crap while still being careful not to spill his pills.

New Grad is sweet enough to come and help me without having to even be asked. I tell her to be careful of her shiny new Dansko shoes because piss can take the shine right out of them and that would be a huge waste of the $220 her grandma spent on them. She asks how I knew her grandma bought them, and I say, "Just a hunch."

Tim is 78 years old and is on a BiPAP machine. This is a machine that has an uncomfortable mask that covers your nose and mouth and literally forces air into your lungs to open your airway enough to oxygenate your blood. Patients' biggest complaint with this is the pressure it creates on the bridge of your nose. He has been here for 13 days on this, and he is getting grumpy and sick of it.

Trust me, Tim. We are sick of it too. Mostly sick of you PISSING IN YOUR WATER CUP, but yeah.

So, I put my armful of crap down and stand there with my hands on my hips. "What in tarnation is happening, Tim? Why? Why do you keep doing this? Don't you see the water in there already??"

I have to literally yell because my N95 mask and his BiPAP machine make it very difficult to communicate.

He just looks at me and shrugs. I say firmly but with love, "That's not an answer, sir. I need to understand why you keep doing this!"

He looks around and tries to speak. I cannot understand him for the life of me because of his BiPAP, so I disconnect it from his face for a second, and he says, "I just had to go really bad."

I immediately replace his mask because his oxygen level has already dropped to 90%, and I try realllllyyy hard not to roll my eyes at him. I know that chronic low oxygen levels can create confusion-like mind states, but damn.

New Grad and I change his gown and the entire bedding and mop the piss-water off the floor with towels that don't even hold liquid anymore because they have been washed so many times. They are so abrasive they'd do better at scrubbing pots and pans than a Brillo pad.

I disconnect his BiPAP again and have him take his pills, which he does quickly so I can hook him back up. I'm hoping to trial him off the BiPAP later today, but I don't have time right now. His assessment is mostly normal, but I can still hear the rattle of the junk in his lungs, even over the machine noise.

New Grad sweetly tidies the room and makes sure his call bell is in reach as she lowers his bed. Once this labor of love is finally complete, I am yet again drenched in sweat. *Have I even had one sip of water yet?*

New Grad and I peel our garbage bags off and walk into the sweet not-so-fresh air of the hallway together. She puts her hand on my shoulder, nods, and takes off. I can tell she is still reeling from her phone call with that family.

I wish I could tell her that it gets easier and doesn't hurt so much over time, but that's not exactly true. It becomes second nature, to live in these terrible moments with people, and then just move on with your day. You become more tolerant of despair. Of pain. Of loss. But believe me when I tell you, you never forget. Not the hard ones. They weigh on your mind and soul every day. This one will cut New Grad deep forever. I know because I have been there. I remember my first code on my patient like it was yesterday.

Walking down the hallway, I'm looking at my handheld, trying to triage who I should give meds to next, when I hear another call for help. I snap out of it and head toward the room where the voice is calling from—a room that isn't mine.

The patient is falling onto the floor beside their bed in a total panic as Dee is trying to keep them from hitting their head. Shit! I gown up quickly and think what an enormous pain in the ass this is, and how people across the country have got to be dying or getting hurt because it takes so damn long to get dressed to go into the rooms.

I run in and help her stabilize the patient without even tying my gown and grab a pillow to put under his head. I call for his nurse, and the three of us somehow get the patient back into bed, but damn. Trying to heave a grown human being off the ground is not an easy task, yo. Luckily this guy could help us a little bit and we managed it. No major injuries, loss of consciousness or new pain, thank you Jesus.

Dee says she was walking by the room and saw him standing by his bedside with his bed alarm going off, all disoriented. Thank God for CNAs. She probably saved this guy from permanent brain damage. Or at least a really bad headache.

9:40 AM

Now what? Oh shit, it's 9:40 and I still haven't given two of my patients their meds yet.

They have to be given before 10:00 am or I have to write up this whole stupid report as to why my patient's medications were late.

Well, Joint Commission, how about you come and do this job and see how many days you are able to perfectly and ideally administer your seven patients' multiple medications while simultaneously making sure no one falls, or dies, or has a stroke, or needs a blanky, or needs water, or has shit themselves, or has a question about their hemorrhoids, or needs to be repositioned, or needs one of the other 792 things on a nurse's list of tasks in one shift?

I will sit behind the nurses' station with my legs crossed at the ankles in my high heels and pencil skirt and sip my iced coffee and take notes while I watch you do this as perfectly and timely as you are demanding of us all.

I'll happily wait; it'll be worth it.

Anyways, I go into the med room and pull Ron's medication out of the Pyxis. He is in room 113 and is the one with the colossal amount of COVID diarrhea, all day every day. This poor man has been dehydrated and super sick for a long time. His ass is so raw, I cannot even tell you. We have put a rectal tube in him three times, and it leaked around it every time, which defeats the purpose, so we have just stopped trying.

Honestly, he should be in the ICU, but because he is not vented (on a ventilator machine), he doesn't qualify nowadays. He has been on continuous BiPAP for 19 days. His oxygen goes into the 50s without it, which is not super compatible with life ... so it stays on. His poor nose is purple and broken down from the pressure of the mask. I've tried every intervention I can think of to relieve the pressure, but there is only so much you can do because you have to maintain a good seal so he can breathe.

The full-face mask doesn't work because he says it hurts his head too much. We have been putting off intubating him because there are no ICU beds available.

None in the entire state.

So ... BiPAP it is.

He's maxed out at 100% oxygen on the BiPAP, he's on multiple medications—most of which are IV—and he needs a new IV bag of fluids. I pull all of his meds from the Pyxis and gown and glove and enter his room.

He is very lethargic and pale. He hasn't eaten in three days and no matter what I do, I cannot get him to take a bite. He's on the list to get a feeding tube inserted, but there are so many critically ill patients in the hospital who need one that the few nurses certified to do it cannot keep up.

I'm going to just have to put a temporary nasogastric (NG) tube in him if they can't do the full CORTRAK soon.*

I set my crap down and start setting up his IV meds on the pumps. I spike the bag and set up his fluids. On physical assessment, I can hear his bowels working overtime even though there is nothing in his system.

He pulls up his mask and takes his couple of pills in one swig, which feels like such a blessed skill. He quickly pulls the mask back in place because the BiPAP alarm goes off in no time without it on.

I ask him how he feels. "Like shit," he says.

I can relate to that. This is not just a metaphorical description, it's also physically accurate. *Well done, Ron. Well done.*

I finish pushing all his IV meds and he's all set up. Ron is my "easy" patient. Very sweet, doesn't ask for anything, just needs help getting cleaned up when he has an episode of diarrhea. He wishes he could control it, but there is no way this amount of shit is controllable—even by someone with impeccable sphincter control.

I check him, and he is miraculously dry. I put his call bell on his chest and ask him to please let me know if he needs anything at all. In this instance, I actually mean it.

9:53 am. *CAN I DO IT??? YES, I CAN!!!* I literally jog to

---

* CORTRAK 2 Enteral Access System, a specialized device used to guide and confirm the placement of feeding tubes.

the med room where, by the grace of the nursing gods (who must have taken off their headphones) there is no line. I log in and take out Barbara's medications in room 111. I am determined to get into that room and scan these meds before 10:00 if it kills me.

Luckily, she only has seven meds, so I pull them out, jog back down the hallway, gown and glove, and get in there. As SOON as I am in the room, my phone rings. I pick it up, and it is Jerry asking for more painkillers.

I start giving Barb her meds, and I tell him I will be with him in a moment, but that I am with another patient right now. He says, "Are you serious right now?" and hangs up on me. *How kind.*

Barb's meds are mostly based on her COVID and lung cancer. Barb is not going to live. She is 88 and has been treated for lung cancer for two years. Her immune system is basically shot. She is rapidly declining. We have been putting off intubating her for days now because we know that she will not live once she is put on a vent.

But interestingly, despite her frail state, she is a full code — that is, we will do everything possible to resuscitate her in the event of cardiac or respiratory arrest. I mean, doing CPR on an 88-year-old, fragile, cancer-ridden patient with no immune system sounds like a brilliant idea to me, so why not, eh?

I have a family meeting scheduled via Zoom today at 11 with our palliative care doctor to try to explain the seriousness of her prognosis. We have tried several times with the family, but they do not want to accept how sick she is. We have been mostly dealing with her daughters, and it's been tough. All I can do is hope and pray that she does not code in the meantime, but it wouldn't be the first time I've broken an old lady's ribs.

Meds are scanned and administered by 9:59. *Damn, I am good.*

I do a gentle assessment, avoiding any unnecessary movements that might increase her already ever-present pain. I make sure Barb has everything she needs and is comfortable.

She says she is in pain and would like some medicine. Taking my garbage bag off, I go back into the med room, get the medication, put a new garbage bag on, and go back in to give it to her.

She closes her eyes and thanks me as I slowly back out of her room while I take off my garbage bag and turn down her lights.

God, I hope her family makes the right choice and listens to her wishes and lets her go. She is technically not able to make her own decisions because of how sick and confused she is, so it's in their hands now.

As I'm rubbing alcohol sanitizer into my hands and standing in the hall, I hear an IV pump go off. I know it's Mildred's vancomycin finishing, so I head down the hallway to switch it back to her primary.

Before I take two steps, her call light goes on. Joy. My favorite sound. I get to her room, and she says, "My IV is beeping."

No shit, Mildred. As if I can't hear the incessant beeping right next to my skull. I'm so happy for you to remind me within five seconds of it starting.

I swallow my sarcasm and switch the pump back to the primary and remove the vanco bag. She tells me her daughter wants to know which medications she is on, and wants me to call her to tell her, and while I'm at it to print her out a list so she can see what they are too. This is very annoying because I know that Theresa has access to our healthcare portal. But, whatever....

On my way to do this, a hospitalist doc stops me in the hall. He is asking about Roxy's episode this morning and wants to know how she is doing now. I tell him she is better, but that I think we need to change her sliding scale because she keeps bottoming out and I've had to give her glucagon five times in four days. I also remind him about the hypotension that I had reported in my text, and explain that I think she needs more fluids and that her kidney failure is probably getting worse. I recommend some bloodwork.

He agrees with all my suggestions and goes to his computer to put the orders in himself.

LOL. Just kidding.

He tells me to put the orders in and he will sign them when he gets a chance. Add this to my list of fuckery. I stand at a computer station, print Mildred's medication list, and go to get it from the printer.

For effing real? It needs toner. *Why me, dude?* One of these days something like this is going to set me over the edge. I go to the storage room and grab a new toner and put it in the printer. It starts printing one million things it had backlogged, so I decide to go do something else while I wait.

I sit down at the nurses' station to document at least a tiny bit of what I need to. I start with entering the new orders for Roxy so that pharmacy can get them and start preparing her meds. I then pick up my personal phone and send my husband a good-morning text and tell him that someone has already died today.

He is an ICU nurse and has been for twelve years. He is incredibly smart, and it is so nice to be with someone who can totally relate to what I do for a living and does it to an even higher degree. He instantly texts back a good-morning response and that he wishes I was snuggled next to him. *SAME.*

I hear the printer stop and go get the medication list I've been waiting on.

I call Theresa and have an extensive conversation about her

mother's medications. It takes 20 minutes of my precious time. I bring the printout to Mildred's room, gown and glove, and go in to hand it to her. I say, "If you or your daughter have any more questions, let me know."

In this instance, I do not actually mean this, and I pray she does not, in fact, let me know about anything at all. Ever.

Heading back to the nurses' station, I sit down again. It's 10:40, so I am hoping to chart for 15 minutes before my Zoom call with Barb's family. I document Roxy's episode this morning, the new orders, and update her vitals, and actually get it finished. I then go into Jerry's chart and am sure to quote him directly with his verbal abuse and assholery. Not that anything will ever be done about it.

Even if I went to management or upper management about it, they would essentially tell me to piss off and—unless he actually put his hands on me—that I better suck it up and accept it's part of my job. I must be empathetic, they would say, to a patient's "suffering" and to the fact that they are in the "most difficult time of their life" since they are in a hospital.

In my opinion, if you are verbally abusing a nurse or medical professional you should be fired from that establishment. Even when patients physically assault us, unless there is a mark or major injury, we are encouraged to brush it under the rug most of the time. I wonder what a hospital CEO would do if a person spoke to them at work like Jerry speaks to me?

By the time I'm done, it's time for my Zoom call. I wish so so so so so much that we could go back to the old days and just meet face to face with these people. Meetings over technology about the literal fate of a loved one seem so callous and inappropriate. And the worst part is being in the room with the patient and having to show the family the state of their loved one over a screen.

I have noticed, though, that it is much less powerful to see your sick and dying loved one through a screen than in person. This has, for example, made some family members less likely to sign off on end-of-life decisions or DNRs (Do Not Resuscitate orders). This is a serious problem—especially in cases like Barb's where she will definitely not survive regardless of whether all interventions are done or not.

I am thankful that the palliative care doc will be on the call today, and just as I am thinking this, I see her walking down the hall.

She looks at me, nods her head, and starts heading to Barb's room. I grab the iPad, start launching Zoom as I walk down the hall, and we stop at the door to get our garbage bags on.

She asks how Barb is doing. I tell her not great, that she is really struggling with every breath and is heavily medicated for comfort and breathing. I explain my worries about her having to be resuscitated or worked up in any way given her frailty and comorbidities, and she agrees. She is Team "Pro-Comfortable Death," and I am so appreciative of this.

Zoom is open, and I look up the family's number on my handheld and text them the Zoom invite. They join the meeting immediately, clearly anxious for the call.

We walk into the darkened room, and I turn on the lights so the family can see her. These lights seem so damn harsh and awful at times like this. Barb's eyes open and adjust to the light. As soon as she sees her family on the screen, she starts to tear up.

Her husband of 67 years, and all four of her kids are on the call, crowding their heads into the screen so she can see that they are all there.

I hate this so much.

The palliative doc starts talking and basically gives a rundown of Barb's hospital stay, and that she is not getting better. As she speaks, Barbara closes her eyes and silently weeps. Every one of her family members is crying, too.

The doc says that Barb has made it known that she is ready to die and would like to do so comfortably and—if possible—at home. She says that unfortunately because of the number of medications she is on, and given her baseline confusion because of her low oxygen, the hospital is mandated to put this final decision on the family because she is not technically "competent" to do so for herself.

Barb's daughters look at her husband and tell him it's up to him. He grabs the screen and brings his face really close as if he is leaning into her. His sweet, hooded, wise old man eyes trying to make eye contact with her. He says shakily, "Look at me, sweet love."

Barb opens her eyes and looks at him through her tears. He declares, "I will do anything you want, especially if it means I get to see you before you go."

She whispers, "Get me home. . . ."

He backs the camera up so the whole family is visible again and says with confidence, "Sign her up for hospice and . . . get her home as soon as you can."

The doc states that this means she will become a DNR immediately, and hospice will be contacted, and she will be brought home via ambulance as soon as all the equipment is delivered. This can be trickier than you'd think, so the doc says we will do our very best to get orders and everything in line right away so she can get her bed and oxygen and medications fast enough that she can go home today.

There is palpable relief in everyone's faces and body language, mine included. Barb stops crying and has a resolve in her face. I'm sure it feels so nice in her brain knowing she will be headed home soon.

I can't believe I didn't cry. That's pretty messed up.

Everything is so completely out of whack and weird. I've made so many of these Zoom calls that they all kind of blur together. I've lost track of how many family members I've watched on a screen say goodbye to a loved one that has been in their lives for many decades.

Or watched as a daughter says goodbye to the single mom who raised her and has always been by her side.

Or as a dad says goodbye to his only son.

On a fucking *screen*.

I truly believe that the risk of getting COVID would be worth seeing your wife of 65 years before she dies, I really do, but again, who am I to make those decisions? I'm just a nurse. I think it should be left up to the family members if they are willing to risk seeing their loved one or not. I do not think that the government or hospital policies should dictate this. I wonder how Joe Biden would feel sitting at home on a computer that he cannot even operate, saying goodbye to his lovely Jill? Or how about Fauci doing this to anyone he loves (if he is even capable of love . . .)?

Honestly, we are lucky that the hospice in town is even taking patients at this point.

11:30 AM

It's 11:30 and I grab my water bottle to take my first glorious sip of stale water from yesterday because I haven't even had time to rinse it out and fill it up again. As I'm doing this, my work phone rings. It's surgery. They tell me that the very kind and understanding Jerry will be going down for surgery at twelve and needs to have a "nose-to-toes" done immediately.

A nose-to-toes is basically a sponge bath in disinfectant. The wipes have a chemical called HCG in them, which kills a bunch of microbes to decrease the chances of a surgical infection. It must be done in a certain order—starting with the head and down to the feet—and cannot be done more than six hours before a procedure.

I mean, I have nothing else to do, so why not? Badging into the storage room, I grab the kit and gown-up to head into his room. He is a very large man, and I have less than 30 minutes to get this done.

I walk in and he is still on his phone playing Mahjong. While I start opening the packages, I explain that I have to do this wipe bath thingy and why. He doesn't even look up from his phone.

I say, "Jerry, I'm going to need you to put your phone down, so I know you are hearing me . . ."

He rolls his eyes and puts his phone on the bedside table. I ask him if he knows what his surgery is for, and he says, "To fix my pain because obviously you can't do it."

"Yes, it's for your abdominal pain, which is being caused by diverticulitis," I explain.

Doing my best to educate him despite my irritation, I tell him that there is a chance that he will come out of surgery with a colostomy.*

He shrugs it off, "The doctor told me she would do everything she could to make sure that doesn't happen. . . ."

I sigh and tell him that he needs to be mentally prepared for the worst because it can be much more difficult to wake up with a colostomy bag when you aren't expecting it.

I pull out my phone and tell him all about online support groups and YouTube videos he could watch to prepare himself while he waits for surgery. When I try to show him an example,

---

* A colostomy is the surgical rerouting of your bowels through a hole on the front of your abdomen. Your bowel movements come out of the whole into a bag adhered to your skin. This can be permanent or temporary and is, unsurprisingly, often a very difficult situation for patients to deal with.

he won't even look at the phone in my hand. He shrugs me off completely, so I give up and finish the wipe bath in silence.

Thank God he can still move reasonably well, and I don't need help turning him.

It's 11:55 now . . . they should be up to take him any minute. I take my drenched garbage bag off and leave the room.

It's basically noon and I haven't done Roxy's 11:30 glucose check yet. Standing in front of the PPE drawers at her room, I see a tiny sticky note on top of the metal container. It reads, "11:30 BGL—246, <3 Dee."

OMG. I love her so much.

I grab the sticky note and head into the med room. 246 mg/dL is a really high blood glucose level, and the sliding scale calls for 10 units of insulin. I get nervous. This is a lot and Roxy is so brittle . . . it makes me anxious, but I have no choice.

Grabbing an insulin syringe, I draw it up in the med room and head to her room, gown up and head in.

She is resting in bed with her high-flow nasal canula on. When I tell her that she needs 10 units of insulin, she starts to look as anxious as I feel. I reassure her that if she starts feeling funny again, she can press her call light, and I will be right with her. She nods and pulls up her gown so I can give her the injection in her front thigh. I scan her wristband and the medication into my handheld, and then uncap the needle. She winces at the pinch of the needle going into her skin. I walk across the room and put the needle in the sharps container. It is full, so that's awesome.

Pulling out my phone, I call EVS to see if someone can come and change out the sharps container. While its ringing, I say goodbye to Roxy, put the call bell on her chest, and remind her to call if she feels weird. She nods her head as an EVS guy answers the phone. He says he will send someone to the floor as soon as possible, and I thank him.

I cannot imagine how busy they are right now; they are evidently down about 50% of their staff because everyone is quitting for higher-paying jobs that deal with less shit. Can't blame them. I take my garbage bag off and wipe down my phone with one of the famous purple sani-wipes.

I walk by room 110, and Jerry is still in there on his dumb phone. Looking down at my watch, I see it's 12:14. *WTF, yo?* I ask the unit secretary if anyone from surgery has called about him, and she shakes her head no. I poke my head in the door and ask him if anyone has been by and he says no. He goes on to try to bad-mouth the hospital, and I just close the door.

Enough is enough, ya know?

Opening the door to Juan's room, before I can ask if I he wants some lunch, I notice that he is playing with his own shit in his hand.

"Someone please grab me a whole bed change and a bunch of towels please?" I say loudly over my shoulder as I gown and glove and attempt to make him stop playing in his own feces. Usually a sweet guy, he is so confused that he is getting violent and tries to kick me when I approach his bed.

No sir, not today. Not any day, but especially not today.

He is screaming at me to leave him alone and screaming for his wife, wanting to know where he is and what we are doing to him. It is too early for sundowning . . . what the hell is going on?*

I speak in a very calm voice and reassure him that I'm here to help, and that his wife loves him very much and will be here soon—which is a lie, but wtf do you want from me? He is covered in his own shit, and I don't want it on me! My backup

---

* Sundowning is when people with dementia or Alzheimer's disease become more confused, agitated, or anxious in the late afternoon, evening, or at night.

Rita finally comes in dressed in her own garbage bag, and I put a blanket over his hands and try to wipe off some of the poop.

"Oh wow . . . that's a lot of poop, Juan," Rita says.

"Yeah . . . this was a good one. . . . " I respond and manage to get the majority off of him in one determined swipe with the blanket.

He is still trying to kick at me and Rita, but we are stronger than we look and eventually are able to wrestle him while cleaning him up and get him back into bed. I call the doc at bedside and ask for a temporary restraint order because Juan is putting himself in danger with his impulsiveness and has a very high risk of serious complications or death if he falls. Plus, it creates a lot of paperwork.

The doc agrees and gives the order for soft wrist restraints and all four bed rails to be up. We press the call button and ask for someone to bring us the restraints. Once we get them, I make sure his wrists are tied firmly but not too tight, put his call bell under his left hand, turn off his lights, and go to get him some medication. He has a prescription for as needed (PRN) lorazepam (Ativan), a benzodiazepine sedative, and I'm using that shit.

Still yelling, he now wants to know why he can't move his arms, but no amount of explaining will help reorient him.

Rachel finishes cleaning up the room while I degown and go get the medication. I find another nurse to witness the disposal of the extra medication and waste one mg of the two-mg syringe (since the order is only for one mg and we have to safely discard the rest because it's a controlled substance).

I gown back up, go into the room, and administer the medication via IV.

Within three minutes he is starting to chill out, so I tidy up a little bit, readjust his position, put his TV on Fox News (his favorite channel), and walk out with Rita.

Good lord. We do inspections of each other and have miraculously come out of that situation with no shit on our scrubs. *WIN*.

I sit down to do some charting because at this point it is 1:00 pm and I have charted close to nothing. I have another phenomenal sip of my stale water and eat a stale graham cracker with peanut butter on it that I stole from the nutrition room. *Awesome.*

As I type, I hear Juan screaming at the top of his lungs, "GET THIS SHIT OFF ME!!!" and can hear the bed rails being rattled around by his arms and legs. I get up and stand in the doorway, watching him through the window as he just loses his ever-loving mind again.

Ativan, you have disappointed me.

But 1 mg of lorazepam is not a lot, so this isn't surprising. I wonder if doctors were nurses, would they ever even bother with a 0.5–1-mg dose of lorazepam for an aggressive patient? I would say, nine times out of ten, it essentially does nothing. I wonder—if they were the ones actually in the rooms having to deal with literal and metaphorical shit like this—if they wouldn't just be like, "TEN MILLIGRAMS STAT!"

My sweet Juan from this morning has become a monster before my eyes. I am standing there with my arms crossed, watching him from the window in the door and, all of a sudden, he starts to get quiet. I unfold my arms and put my hands on my hips because this is probably not a good sign. Watching his vitals monitor, I see his oxygen saturation steadily decrease . . . 95% . . . 93% . . . 92% . . . 90%. . . .

The hair on the back of my neck stands up, and I get a terrible feeling in my gut . . . 88% . . . 87% . . . *fuck.*

I start gowning up and yell to Emma to page respiratory therapy stat and call a rapid response. His BP is tanking too—currently 93/76. Jesus. I go in the room and try to arouse him by calling his name. He barely opens his eyes and starts to breathe all irregularly and way too fast.

Shit, this is bad.

His heart rate is okay at 72; I change the settings on the monitor to recheck blood pressure every two minutes, and the cuff starts going again. His oxygen is somehow holding steady at 83%.

I hear the rapid response being called on the overhead paging system and wait for the rush of humans into the room. I hear that dumb squeaky wheel of the code cart out in the hallway and know Emma is getting it ready just in case. Next, I hear garbage bags rustling outside of the door as I am trying to keep Juan with me. He is squeezing the shit out of my hand. Normally I would be running around like an idiot getting all the meds and everything I could possibly need for a total shitshow, but because of COVID, I'm just chilling in my garbage bag holding the hand of this man who just moments ago was trying to kick me.

The door opens, and a bunch of other garbage bags walk in and start hooking him up to machines. Emma chucks a bunch of IV supplies at me, and I start trying to get another IV line. They get an EKG to measure his heart rhythm, phlebotomy comes in to draw STAT labs, respiratory therapy gets him set up on BiPAP, and I start asking the doc what he wants me to do about his low blood pressure at 82/64.

Oxygen saturation is now hovering at 78%, and he is only responding to painful stimuli like a sternal rub.

We hook him up to the BiPAP and put 100% oxygen on for him; meanwhile the doc wants Levophed hung (started as an IV drip) because his next BP is 78/59. Levophed is a quick-acting and powerful blood pressure-supporting medication that is given to sustain life for critically low BP. In most cases, it is technically life support.

I tell him we don't run that drip down here on the medical floor, only the ICU does it.

He tells me, "I don't care, make it work."

I look at my charge nurse, Ryan, who is in here helping, and he shrugs and says let's do it and dials the ICU on his phone. He begs them for a bed. The news is good, "Great, as soon as the room is clean, he needs to be up there. We are maxed on BiPAP and starting levo."

I bet someone just died up there. That's why the room's available.

We literally do not even have Levophed down here, so I call my girl Tara who works up in the ICU and ask her to pull me a bag. I look at Dee the CNA, meet her eyes and ask her to please run up to the ICU and grab it since I don't want to leave him. She nods, quickly degowns and jogs down the hallway.

I start a bolus of LR fluid in the new IV that I got in his right bicep and put it wide open, hoping it will help his BP. Someone is putting on the shock pads and CPR monitoring system just in case shit really goes downhill. His heart rate is now 165 but is so far normal ("sinus") rhythm.

The doc starts asking me a bunch of history questions on him and wants to know what the likely cause of this episode is. My gut tells me it's the COVID that's made him generally unstable, and with his dementia, he wasn't able to let us know that he felt extra bad this morning.

Suddenly, he goes unresponsive and into ventricular fibrillation (V-fib), which is a heart rhythm not conducive with life.

God damn it, Juan.

The doc orders a synchronized cardioversion. This means that they will shock him, but the machine will do it in sync with his heart rhythm as it is. The goal is to basically turn the power button of the heart off and right back on again—a reset—to make it work right again.

I turn the knob on the defib monitor to "synchronized," and Emma draws up some midazolam (Versed) and fentanyl for a little sedation/pain control because this shit hurts. She hands it to me, and I push them both pretty fast because I know that they will cardiovert ASAP. The monitor says it's synchronized, and the doc gives the go ahead, so I loudly say "CLEAR!" and everyone backs off with their hands in the air.

(Yes, it's really like in the movies.)

One of the other garbage bag people presses the shock button, and his heart stops and then restarts. Right back into V-fib. He has a pulse but remains unresponsive. Amiodarone—a powerful drug used to try to correct the heart rhythm—is drawn up and administered per MD orders, and I am prepping for another synchronized shock, when he goes into asystole and we lose a pulse. I immediately kneel on the side of the bed and start compressions.

Someone pushes the code blue button. There's about to be 1,000 residents and interns and a whole critical care team up in here, and it already feels like there's 50 people in this tiny room. I am legitimately overheating in this garbage bag outfit, and doing compressions with an N95 mask on can suck my balls.

After two minutes, a pulse check is ordered. I stop doing compressions so it can be checked, but no pulse is found. More people come rushing into the room, but most just stand outside the door because administration has been pushing to have fewer people in the COVID rooms during codes to prevent the spread of the infection.

One of the male nurses, John, takes over doing compressions, and I can hear the recorder—the team member who documents all interventions, timings, and medications during CPR—and docs shouting out times and meds to be administered. We are on round two of epinephrine, sodium bicarbonate's already been given, amiodarone is being drawn up, and now we just continue to do compressions until we get a pulse. Or not.

One of the fellows (the ones above "residents") attempts to intubate him but misses the first time. He ends up getting it the second time, the ambu-bag is hooked up to his endotracheal tube (breathing tube), and air from the bag is forced into his lungs each time the respiratory therapist squeezes it. This allows us to get his oxygen level back up to normal much faster than without an artificial airway.

It is so gross to watch someone be intubated—you can literally see the hard plastic deform their throats as it's pushed unnaturally down into the lungs. It grosses me out every time.

Mother of God it is hot AF in here....

Everyone in here is sweating like its monsoon season. Ryan tells anyone who is not actively doing something to get out of the room.

We are on round five of compressions, and my forearms and shoulders and core are all burning. Don't have to go to the gym later, at least. My gloves are gross and full of sweat, and I am trying so hard not to think about them.

We pause for another pulse check: nothing. Someone rotates compressions with me, and I don't even know who they are. Probably a new resident or something.

Juan, this is not generally a good direction to keep going in.

Compressions are immediately resumed, and epinephrine is pushed yet again. We do this cycle: two minutes of compressions, pulse check, epinephrine every other time, compressions, pulse check, until we all die along with Juan.

I vaguely hear the recorder say it's been 34 minutes, and I look at the doc and beg him through my COVID goggles to stop. This poor man. I know for a fact that I've broken multiple ribs, or at least cracked the shit out of his cartilage, and I don't even legitimately know how he could possibly live even if we did by some miracle get a pulse back. Doc calls it, and I gratefully get down off the bed and stop doing compressions.

Time of death: 13:56.

2:00 PM

We all stand there in a quiet moment of "We're sorry . . . we did the best we could," which is done every time a person dies in this way.

Unlike on TV, it's rare that a healthcare professional loses their shit and throws their gloves off onto the floor while storming away because the patient died. If they did, I would follow them into the hallway and point back in the room and say, "YOU DROPPED SOMETHING," very aggressively until they cleaned up their mess.

The doc starts reviewing how the code went, what we should have done differently, anything we could have possibly missed, and what we did very well. No one has any ideas what we could have done better—this was just a shit situation.

What a total whirlwind.

I ask if the Ativan I gave him could have caused this, and the docs all say no, they believe this was a totally separate issue. Living through things like this really puts life into perspective. While the doc is talking, I am unhooking Juan from all he machines and monitors that were emergently placed all over his body. I clean up wrappers and flushes and syringes and gauze and various other things from the bed.

Closing Juan's eyes, I say a quiet blessing to him and release his soul. Everyone walks out of the room except me and Emma. Still trash bags. Still sweating. Still here. I change my gloves because, *ewww*.

We start to clean Juan up and prepare his body for the morgue.

This entails cleaning up his urine and feces from the pressure placed on his body from coding. We keep all his IVs in because he will be a coroner's case since his death was not planned and he has COVID. (Did you know dead bodies still bleed from holes in their skin? Sometimes A LOT.)

We start chatting about our lives. Emma tells me about this boy she likes, but that he talks to a bunch of other women, and it hurts her feelings. I am taking all the EKG stickers off Juan's bare chest while I tell her that she deserves to be the entire center of a man's world and screw that guy. She is taking all the IV fluids and tubing out of the pumps to throw them away and laughs over the sound of all the beeping and says something about how it's easier said than done.

I nod and say I know, but that she is an effing gem, and I'll kick the shit outta that guy for being a dick and treating her like she's average. I say this as I roll Juan's limp body over so that she can clean him, wipe him down, and place a new chuck pad under him for in the body bag.

"You're a nutcase, Tiffany," she says, while we roll him over to her side and I take all the dirty linen out from under him and roll the clean ones out. We both laugh and finish cleaning up his front while bantering about me kicking the shit out of asshole men. I brush his hair, center the cross necklace he is wearing, and hold his hand for a second—it's already starting to turn blue.

Once his body is ready, Emma grabs the white body bag kit. I label it and we both sign the tag that goes on his toe (yes this is done in real life) and the actual bag itself. We have to double-bag him because of COVID, so we put another bag inside the signed one. I roll him to my side, she sticks one side of him in the bag, then we roll him the other way and put the other side in.

While we work, we haven't had to communicate a single word about what we are doing . . . unfortunately, we have become absolute pros at this bagging a body thing.

I call transport to let them know we have a body for the morgue, and they say they are on their way. We finish cleaning up the room, emptying the trashes, emptying the linen bag, wiping everything down.

I mean truly, when I went to nursing school, this seemed so much more glamorous than it really is. I had this picture that if my patient were dying, I would be sitting with perfect posture and perfect hair in a chair next to them, holding their hands, with a glimmering tear rolling down my face, telling them that it'll be okay, while their loved ones looked on and were in awe of my amazing nursing abilities. And then when they die, I kiss their forehead, walk out of the room and call someone else to deal with "the rest."

LOL. I AM the rest.

We are done, so we leave and shut the door, and Emma walks away to go check on her people because we have been in there for quite a while. I print the needed paperwork for the morgue and put it on the cart outside his room.

It's 14:43. Standing in the hall, I feel like it is a different day from this morning when I went into Juan's room and held his hand.

I must release him and not allow this to affect my entire day. I close my eyes and take two deep breaths. The toughest part is yet to come, dealing with the poor family's grief. Maybe they will be satisfied with the call from the doctor. Doc walks by me and says he already called the wife, and she would like me to call with more details.

Shit.

As I'm walking to the nurses' station, I glance into room 110 and still see Jerry laying in his bed on his phone. *NOOOOOOOO*. He isn't in surgery . . . and I smell shit in the air . . . *UGHHH*. If he has shit himself, I'll have to redo the nose-to-toes.

I try to get by his doorway without making eye contact and am successful thanks to the exciting nature of whatever BS he is watching on his phone (which I am certain is not the educational stuff I recommended). As I approach the desk, the unit secretary looks at me and rolls her eyes and says that Jerry has been real aggro about the fact that he's not in surgery and has been incredibly demanding while I was in coding Juan.

Are you for real?

I call down to pre-op to ask *wtf the hold up is, yo?* And the nurse says, "Yeah sorry, we had an emergent gunshot wound surgery that we had to move in front of his since we only have the one general surgery team on today."

Perfect. Gunshot wound. The world is just such a fantastic place, I can't even begin to tell you.

To avoid gowning up, I walk up to Jerry's door and poke my head in. As soon as I do, he starts bitching about how long it's been since he's seen me. I tell him that someone just passed away, and he mumbles something about how if this hospital can't handle both dying people and the other people on the floor, then they shouldn't be open at all.

"What did you just say?" I ask.

"Nothing . . ." he mutters under his breath and then asks when he's going down for surgery. I tell him no later than three, and that I'll be back in to clean him up and do another nose-to-toes wipe down, and he starts to lose his mind. I just close the door and walk away. This is becoming a pattern.

I go into the supply room and grab yet another lovely kit to bring to Jerry's room along with new bedding and wipes, and my girl Kirsten is in there. We strike up a conversation, she expresses her sadness about Juan, and I say thanks. She says, "At least he didn't end up having to rot away in a nursing home from his dementia," and I totally agree with that.

Clearly, I am putting off calling his family, but the man is dead, and I need to get this other guy to surgery, or I am super screwed. I ask if she will help me, and she straight-up refuses, "Dude, he can turn himself. Hell no."

Son of a bitch, haha. That would have been my response too, so I'm not even mad. We have a kindred soul relationship . . . we've both been nurses for a while and living through this COVID nonsense has given us an indestructible bond. We also have some similar historical trauma bullshit, so we work well together, to say the least.

I start walking toward room 110, and I can already feel myself beginning to sweat again. After gowning up, I grab my supplies and brace myself for the unleashing of Jerry's toxic mouth. He complains the entire time I am in the room. About me. About the food here. About the TV station availability. About the TV size. About how the CNA won't just literally do anything and everything for him. About the blanket quality (which I will give him this . . . they are BAD). About the view of a brick wall that his room has. That he feels as if we are all very impersonal because of all our personal protective gear for COVID. About the lighting. I swear to God, I couldn't even make this up.

I am incredibly proud of myself because the only noise I make in response is a small grunt of agreement when he talks about the blankets. Otherwise, I keep my big mouth sealed so I don't get my ass fired for saying what I'm actually thinking.

He is so large that turning him in the bed is a challenge. He is up against the rail on both sides with not a single inch to spare, and I do much of the work to get him there. After cleaning up his shit and changing all of his bedding, I start the nose-to-toes rinse down yet again. Once I am done wiping down all his layers and extensive area of skin, I tell him he is done and will be headed down shortly. *Please let it be true.* it might push me over the edge if I have to do that again.

I degown, head out of the room and bump directly into the wound care nurse who is taking care of Mildred. Looks like I'm going to be waiting a little longer to call Juan's family. Hearing a *bing*, I see a text on my work phone that Roxy's blood glucose level is now 534, despite me having given her 10 units of insulin earlier.

What is going on?

I text the doctor and ask what to do. He says she needs an insulin drip. I ask him if that's a good idea considering she's not technically in DKA and she goes hypoglycemic so easily. He thinks about it, and agrees, leaving us without a plan. After some back-and-forth, we agree that she needs hourly glucose checks with a low-end sliding scale that includes an extra five units of insulin if her sugar is over 500. He says he will put the order in because he's sitting at a computer. Thank you, Lord because I am slammed.

It's ten past three, but I should have a few minutes before the order is in the system and approved by pharmacy, so I head down to Mildred's room to help wound care.

On my walk down the hall, I take a moment to appreciate the doctors who look at nurses as coworkers, not subordinates.

Listen, I understand that doctors and nurses are not the same thing, thank you very much. I get that they spend way more time at school than us. But the point is, we have a skill set that they don't. We can do things that they would never even dream of doing, and vice versa. This is what makes us COWORKERS, and how we should work together as a team.

When a doc like the one I just spoke to takes my advice and

works WITH me and not AGAINST me, not only can it save time, but it can truly saves lives. We all have to catch each other and make sure we're making the best decisions and performing the best we can for our patients.

By the time I'm done with my little moment of appreciation, I am gowned and opening Mildred's door. Karrie, our sweet South African wound care nurse, is in the room sweating up a storm trying to get poor Mildred's leg in a position so she can see her heel. Have you ever tried to get an older person laying in bed to raise their leg up high enough that you can see their entire heel area?

I'm here to tell you it's near impossible.

I briskly walk over to the bed and grab ahold of her leg at her knee and ankle. Straightening them out, I raise them so that Karrie can get a good photo for her record.

"Hello, darling, how is your life?" she asks in her sweet South African accent.

I briefly look at her in uncomfortable silence until she looks up at me, and I say, "SO GREAT."

She giggles a little and says, "I'm glad everything is working out so well for you. Shame it couldn't be better."

We both laugh a little. Mildred's entire leg is hiked up into the air like a woman giving birth, but somehow she is sleeping. I have no idea how patients sleep through stuff like this.

Once Karrie gets her pictures, we cover the wound with a simple saline-soaked gauze dressing and an absorbent wound pad and then wrap it with a rolled gauze dressing. Nothing fancy is needed because she will need a surgical debridement or possibly even an amputation.

Almost the instant we have her fully repositioned and covered up and comfortable, the general surgeon walks in the room and asks to look at the foot. Why the hell does this always happen? Timing is everything, people! (I have a momentary thought of, "If this is the only general surgeon on today, why is he up here instead of operating on Jerry?" but decide to mention this later.)

I wake Mildred up because the surgeon needs to speak with her. I call her daughter, Theresa, to get her on speaker phone too because she is her medical proxy and is currently the one responsible for her medical decisions.

Theresa answers with an aggressive "Yes?!"

I introduce myself and the surgeon and tell her that we are in the room with her mom assessing her foot. I take the dressing we literally just put on back off and show the surgeon what it looks like by again hiking poor Mildred's leg into the air.

The surgeon starts talking. "Well, based on the MRI results, X-ray, CT scan, and what I see here, there is really no way to get around amputation of this foot. She will likely need a below-the-knee amputation done sooner rather than later given the extent of this infection and the disease process. I will consult with orthopedics to ensure they agree with my assessment. Given her COVID-positive status, she is at a higher risk of complications such as prolonged intubation, difficulty with anesthesia, respiratory failure, and possible death. Is this a risk you are willing to take, ma'am?"

Theresa starts just absolutely losing her mind over the phone.

"What do you mean she needs an amputation? I sent her in there with a wound and now you're saying amputation?! She's 79 years old and lives in a nursing home! What kind of doctor suggests a 79-year-old woman gets an amputation? She will never walk again!"

The surgeon takes a breath and says, "Ma'am, your mother will definitely not walk again without this surgery. She will also likely die because the infection will keep spreading through her bones and will eventually kill her, even with proper IV antibiotics. If you choose not to have the surgery, then she will need to be placed on palliative care and eventually hospice to manage her comfort and pain. If you choose to allow the surgery, recovery will be tough at her age, yes, but she has a chance of living several more years pain- and infection-free."

There is dead silence on the other end of the phone as Theresa takes in this news. I say, "Are you still there?"

She pipes up, "Of course I am. I just can't imagine that these are our only two options. I'm a nurse practitioner and can think of at least five other options."

The surgeon and I look at each other and he says, "And what may those be?"

Silence again, then, "Long-term antibiotic use for one!" she yells.

Alrighty then, Theresa. Take it down a few pegs. The surgeon stays calm and cool and says "Yes . . . and she will be on long-term antibiotic therapy regardless of the route you choose here. Anything else?"

More silence.

I can tell Theresa is upset, and Mildred pipes up, "I want the surgery, Theresa. Let them do it. It will give me more time."

The surgeon nods his head while Theresa says, "Okay, mom, we will try it. I give consent for the surgery."

The surgeon explains, "I'll have to have the ortho team reach out to get official consent and to schedule her into their books ASAP."

Theresa agrees to this and hangs on to speak more with Mildred. The surgeon degowns and leaves the room and starts to walk away. "Doc?" I call out with gumption, while trying to get out the door fast enough to catch him. He stops in his tracks and turns around. "When will room 110 be going down to see you? I have already pre-oped him twice today and would love it to happen, if possible."

"Yes, he's next on my list, we will call for him within the next 15 minutes. I'm headed to scrub in now."

It's so weird how excited surgeons get when they get to cut someone open.

I regown and head back into Mildred's room. Attempting to escape, I finish up the phone call with Theresa as quickly as humanly possible while wrapping Mildred's foot back up for the second time in 15 minutes. Mildred says goodbye and I love you to Theresa, and I hang up the phone. I tuck Mildred all back in and make her comfortable once again. Karrie had to take off while the surgeon was here because her list of patients is never ending. I make sure Mildred's table, call light, and phone are all within reach. I take her vitals, and everything is normal. I ask her if there is anything else I can get for her, and she says, "No thank you, dear. I guess I'll be having surgery now because of this foot."

I tell her yes, she will, but she will be okay and will adjust to life without her foot. She laughs slightly and says, "Yeah, I suppose I will, won't I?"

I start stripping off layers, dim the lights and walk out of the room, praying she gets a nap.

3:40 PM

I glance at my watch and see that it is 3:40.

I walk by room 110 hesitantly because I think I'll truly lose my mind if Jerry isn't in surgery, but I see that his bed is gone from the room, so I do a mini happy dance in my brain. Not in real life. This gives me a little pep in my step walking to my computer until I realize I have to call Juan's family.

Shit. God, I hate this. I hate COVID. I hate people dying

alone. I hate that this is the second death call I've had to make today and it's not even 4 pm. Being a nurse is my true dharma, as my mom says. It's really what I was put on this earth to do. I usually love it . . . the pace, the service of people, healing people, critical thinking, bantering with coworkers . . . everything!

Except this. I hate this. But I may as well get it over with.

I sit down and log in to the computer and find Juan's wife's phone number. Rosa is her name. *UGH*.

Okay, I dial the number. She picks up right away, "Hello?"

I take a deep breath. "Hi, Mrs. Rodriguez, this is Tiffany, the nurse taking care of Juan, how are you today?"

Straight away, I can hear the air being let out of her lungs as she asks for details of her husband's death that she probably doesn't really want but needs.

"I just wanted to hear from you what happened because the doctor was confusing me."

I close my eyes and say, "Well, Juan started to get very agitated and upset, which can be a sign that either something is wrong, or just that he is upset. I was watching him closely, we had to restrain him at one point because he was trying to hit the staff."

I hear a soft, "Oh my God, I am so sorry," and I continue.

"His blood pressure was very low, and after a while, he was not able to keep his oxygen level up. His heart started to malfunction and went into a rhythm not compatible with life. Once that happened, we had to start CPR on him. We did CPR for a while, but we were not able to bring him back, unfortunately. I am so sorry, Rosa. I know how hard this is."

She is silent. I mean, what do you really say to that? I can hear her crying. She says weakly, "Okay. I just wish I could have seen him one last time."

I know. I really do.

She continues, "You know, with his dementia, he's been mostly gone from me for many years. But he would recognize me most times and his eyes would fill with tears, and he would be so happy just to be near me. I will miss him so much. Thank you for taking care of him."

I tell her it was my pleasure and tell her to call me if she needs anything else. We say our pleasantries and she hangs up. Staring blankly at my screen, so may thoughts are racing through my mind. As if having dementia and being confused and scared all the time isn't bad enough . . . then to get COVID and be isolated and away from everything and everyone that is even remotely routine and familiar?

That's some rough shit, dude.

Dee saunters by with a sticky note in her hand and puts it on my black screen. She also puts an energy drink in front of me because she is my soul sister, and she totally knows I need it. I am eternally grateful for people like her in my life. I hope that when it's my time to die, people like her surround my soul and wrap me in love and send me on my way.

The sticky note says, "Roxy BGL 469." Well, at least it's coming down a little bit. I'll have to address that in a little while, but for now we are going in the right direction.

I get up and make the decision that I am going to finally go pee. I go to the staff bathroom, go to turn the handle, and realize it is locked. *Absolutely perfect.* I go to the next unit down the hall, and by the grace of the Lord it is open.

Sitting down on the toilet, I put my head in my hands. I take some measured deep breaths and feel a buzz in my pocket. I wince as I pull out my work phone and see a message from pharmacy that Mildred's antibiotic dose has been updated and changed based on her lab results. Word. I quickly respond with a thank you and wonder what my life would be like if I chose a different profession.

I look up and there's a bulletin board on the wall with a whole bunch of shit from management about what nurses are doing wrong. There are pictures of patient's wounds that we were held accountable for as hospital-acquired pressure injuries. There are posters about how we need to chart better, do better, and handle more with little smiley face emojis at the end to sweeten the message a bit. There's a little "hospital update" article written by our director of nursing that's full of bullshit and fluff and I suppose is meant to improve morale.

LOL. It's amazing to me that we cannot even shit in peace in this place. *Do more! Do better! Keep track of more and more crap!!!*

I wash my hands, shaking my head at the business of healthcare, and how out of control it has gotten.

Slowly I walk back down the hallway to my unit and do a quick recount of my internal to-do list. I sit down at my charting station and heave a deep breath of stale hospital air into my lungs. I gather my brain and wiggle my mouse to wake up my computer.

The amount of charting that I have to catch up on is literally ridiculous. I log in with my credentials and think for the $7,469^{th}$ time in my head how outrageous the requirements for passwords are nowadays. It's like, a capital letter, a lowercase letter, a number, a special character, and it can't resemble a word or name or have your date of birth in it, and also you should put ancient cave symbols in there, too.

I mean, really.

I log in and start typing my note about Juan's code and death. I go find Ryan, who was the recorder for the code, and ask him where his record is. He literally hands me a paper towel with his chicken scratch on it. I look up at him with huge round eyes, and he goes, "Sorry bro, I haven't had time to transcribe it yet."

Jesus Christ.

Sitting back in my chair and wiggling my mouse to wake the computer, I have to enter my 900-character long password again and start to transcribe this chicken scratch by trying to discern what it says and comparing it with my memory of the event. I think I get most of it right, and then document that postmortem care was done and that I spoke to his wife.

Isn't it so crazy that such life-altering occurrences like preparing a dead body and speaking to their family members about their death can be put into one brief sentence in a note? As if these enormous, incredibly powerful and important moments in people's lives are just an inconsequential blurb on a piece of paper. As if hearing details about how your loved one died is just par for the course. As if telling someone the details of their loved one's death that you were just a part of is not a big deal.

It's so weird, the life of a nurse.

Once I finish that note, I start going through my other patients' charts and begin my notes on them but save them to finish later. I go through and put all my patients' vital sign data into the EMR, look at recent lab results, and notice that I have to replace Tim's potassium because it's only 3.5. I make a mental note to grab a supplement when I get his evening meds. I do some more reading and documenting in charts and am about to start my fourth note when I hear an overhead page, "Nurse to room 113, nurse to room 113."

Damn. I almost got caught up with my paperwork for a second there! I head over to Ron's room and look in the window.

Ughhh, poor guy. I can see the diarrhea on the floor and all over the bed—he is laying as still as possible trying not to make the mess even bigger. Opening his door a crack, I say, "I'm coming as soon as I can, I've gotta grab some supplies."

He just calmly nods his head and waits. I notice he looks a

little gray and say a silent prayer for him. With this amount of diarrhea, I can't believe that he tested negative for *Clostridium difficile*, a dangerous bacterial infection of the gut that causes profuse, watery BMs.

Heading to the supply room, I grab all new bedding, multiple towels, wipes, and a new bottle of soap. I stand there looking at the shelves, trying to make sure I didn't forget anything, and decide I have everything I need. I reach his door, gown and glove, grab my armful of supplies, and head in there.

Turning on all the lights, I put my supplies on the bedside table. He looks at me with tears in his eyes, mouthing through his BiPAP mask that he is sorry. I take a second and hold his hand and look him in the eyes and tell him it is not a problem and that we will get him fixed up right away.

Normally, he is able to help me with this and can turn himself from side to side and stay sitting up so I can get him clean and the bed changed. Today, though, he is hardly able to shift his weight. Something is off, so I go to the other side of the bed and get down to his level after lowering the bed rail.

I look him in the eyes again and say, "Are you okay? Can you move like usual?" and he just weakly shakes his head that he cannot.

No. He is not dying on me today, that would be far too much death for a real-life nursing shift. Maybe in *Grey's Anatomy*, three patients die in one shift, but not in real life. He is clearly struggling to breathe and is just exhausted. I get my phone out and dial the hospitalist doc's extension. No answer. *Typical*. I press the call light and ask for Ryan.

I start getting Ron cleaned up. A few minutes later, Ryan pokes his head into the room. "What's up?" he says.

I sigh, "He's decompensating and tuckering out—I'm not sure how much longer he has on this BiPAP, and he is also severely dehydrated because of this never-ending diarrhea. I need the doc in here asap if you could please get him."

He nods his head and leaves.

Even though I have to do most of the work this time, I get Ron all cleaned up and with a fresh blanket and gown and stand there holding his hand until the doc comes in the room.

Ron is a really gray complexion now and is breathing about 40 breaths per minute, which is way too fast, and is using his "accessory muscles," rib cage muscles that are only used on exertional breathing. Not a good sign. He needs to be intubated and put in the ICU.

I give the doc the same update I did to Ryan and tell him I think it's about intubation time. Ron is essentially unconscious and in a deep sleep already. Doc agrees that he needs to go the ICU and to the intubation, but we there are no free ICU beds right now. I asked about the bed from before, during the code, and he said it hasn't been cleaned thoroughly yet.

(Oh yeah, I forgot about the super intense cleaning that has to happen to these rooms after a COVID patient dies in them.)

Okay, so we must wait. The doc suggests maybe flight for life-ing him out to a bigger hospital and says he will make some calls. Nodding, I begin cleaning up the room from the explosion. I clean the shit off the floor with a high-quality towel and then sani-wipe the entire area. I sani-wipe his bed and the bed rails, and everything else that had poop on it. I put all the shit garbage in one garbage can and put all of his dirty linen into the separate linen bag. Once everything is clean and sanitized, I take the garbage and linen bags out, tie them up, and remove my own garbage bag gown and put it in the other can.

I walk out the door and heave the two heavy bags to the soiled linen room. All the receptacles are overflowing with trash and linen. *Lovely*. I am so appreciative of the men and women who take these out all day every day. They are as much part of the medical team as any of us bedside. I can't imagine having to go down to the basement or out to the dumpster every single time I had bags of trash or linen. I wash my hands with actual soap and water in the soiled linen room and grab a paper towel to dry them off.

The smell in here makes my eyes water.

4:15 PM

I briskly walk out of the room and look back through the window. He is just lying there all gray and uncomfortable in the darkness of his room. I say another little prayer.

Looking at my watch, I see it's 4:16 pm. Pulling out my work phone, I look and see that Tim has meds and an IV antibiotic due. I go into the med room, and Kirsten is in there blankly looking at the screen, trying to remember what she's in there for. I recognize that look. She looks up and says, "How are your people? You doing okay?"

"Another day in COVID paradise as usual! But yes, I am okay. You?"

She grumbles something along the lines of "This shit is not paradise," and logs out of the Pyxis and purposefully bumps my shoulder on her way out the door.

I wonder how many times in my career I have both said and heard some form of the phrase "ANOTHER DAY IN PARADISE." It's such a dumb saying. But I'm sarcastic and silly and I think it's ironically funny to say shit like that because this is sooooo sooooo far away from any kind of paradise.

I badge into the Pyxis and put my right middle finger down on the clear glass fingerprint reader. I often use my middle finger to passive-aggressively express my feelings towards this job and I love flipping this thing off multiple times a day.

It tells me my fingerprint is spoofed and can't be read.

WTF. I do it again. Spoofed again. MOTHER EFFER DON'T SET ME OVER THE EDGE, MACHINE!!! Third time is the charm, and it lets me in.

I grab Tim's steroids, potassium supplement, and proton pump inhibitor along with his antibiotics and the 100-mL normal saline bag to mix it in. As I press "log out," Emma walks in the door. She starts telling me about her patient in room 119, who is just not doing well. She just had to have her BiPAP settings increased and nothing we are doing is helping her. She says she hasn't had time to even sit down yet and she's so far behind in her charting that she doesn't even know where to start. Man, can I relate to that!

I ask her what I can do for her and, of course, she says "Nothing." Nurses have an intrinsic inability to ask for help unless we have literally no other choice. I tell her to come get me or call me if she needs anything at all. She nods and badges into the Pyxis.

I walk out into the hallway, and down to room 114. Tim is chilling in his bed watching TV. I gown and glove and go in there, and . . . .*what in the . . . ? Are you serious? THERE IS URINE IN THE URINAL!!! By all the heavens, for all the blessings, THANK YOU GOD!*

I go over to him all excited and say, "Tim!!! You used the urinal!!!"

He nods his head and says through his BiPAP, "I'm a big boy now!"

Hahahaha, I giggle, and it feels nice to have an uplifting conversation for once. I tell him I want to try him off the BiPAP for a little bit. He agrees, and I grab the high-flow nasal canula and switch the BiPAP out with it.

He rubs his nose and sighs in relief and says, "God that thing sucks."

"Actually, it blows, but yeah," I reply.

He laughs to himself a little at my pun and takes his meds after commenting on the enormous horse pill that is potassium supplements. *Why are they so big???*

I mix his IV, scan all the medication labels, scan his wrist band, and hook up his antibiotics. Hooking him up to the oxygen monitor, I see that he is saturating at 92%. He sees this, and I tell him that as long as he is tolerating it and saturating well, we will keep him on the high flow. He raises his hand for a high five, and I of course oblige him. He smiles, and it is a tiny, sweet reward for my heart. I smile back at him under my mask.

I hope he can see it through my eyes.

I note for my charting how much urine was in his urinal (finally!) before emptying it.

Tearing off a garbage bag dress for the thousandth time today, I walk back into the hallway. Walking to the nurses' station to document some more, I'm told by the unit secretary that I have Barb's family on the phone.

Oh shit! I wonder where we are at in the transfer process. I go find the case manager and ask where we stand with getting her home.

He says that we are waiting on confirmation of a hospital bed delivery to their house, but that it has been ordered and accepted by the DME (Durable Medical Equipment) company. Once we have that, we will arrange her transfer by ambulance. I pick up the phone and tell the daughter all this, and she is very thankful for the update, but asks how come she was the one that had to call me.

I apologize for not getting back to her sooner, but she is a little perturbed and says, "Yeah, well I figured since we hadn't heard from you that I better call."

"I'm sorry you've all had to wait, sometimes the day gets away from me. But if anything major changes or transport is arranged, either myself or the case manager will call to let you know."

"Well," she replies, "I guess we will just keep waiting for all of you to get your shit together enough to get my dying mom home."

I roll my eyes instead of saying what I want to, which is, *I have no control over the DME company, the insurance company, or the ambulance company. As soon as I do, the world will be a better place.*

Because I want to keep my job, I say, "Okay, well I hope we are able to meet your expectations shortly because I know how important it is for Barb to get home before she gets much worse."

Her daughter says thanks and hangs up.

I walk over to the case manager and again express how important it is for Barb to get home so that she does not die in this place . . . he nods his head and picks up the phone to call the DME company once again. I wonder what it would be like if everyone involved in these cases were to treat every patient they served like a member of their family.

I mean, if your mom was dying in the hospital, and her last wish was to get home to die with dignity next to your dad, wouldn't you do *everything* in your power to make that happen? The DME companies drag their feet so badly . . . and I know that some of that is insurance—waiting for insurance approval, paperwork, or authorization processes (let's be honest, it's probably almost all insurance)—but it is still so frustrating when there is a sick human being who just needs a hospital bed delivered so she can die in peace.

I stroll down to room 112 while scrolling through my handheld and peek through the window in the door to see sweet Roxy laying in bed with her eyes closed. Her favorite show, *House Hunters* is on her screen, but she is sleeping soundly. I take my time gowning and gloving, as my energy is starting to wane.

It's 4:52 pm, and my brain and heart are worn.

I slowly walk in, but the gorgeous rustling sound my garbage outfit makes wakes Roxy up. She smiles when she sees me and says, "Time for a sugar check?"

I nod and grab the glucometer. This is the most alert and awake I have seen her all day. I grab my badge from under my gown and sign into the machine. Scanning the strips, I then scan her bracelet and poke her finger. She stays still as I put the drop of blood on the strip and wait for the machine to do its magic. 414. Okay! We are slowly but surely getting to where we need to go.

I ask her if she's ordered dinner, and she tells me not yet. I offer to order for her, and she is so happy to accept this offer because waiting on hold with the operating system blows. She lets me know what she wants, and I tell her I will be back with some more insulin and I will put in her order asap.

I degown and deglove and, as I leave, I ask if there is really nothing I can bring her and she shakes her head no. Damn, so rarely is a patient this easy. I get out into the hallway and hear my name on the overhead: "Tiffany to room 113, Tiffany to room 113."

Crap. Ron has shit again, I guarantee it. Poor guy.

I use the alcohol hand sanitizer and walk one door down to Ron's room. *Damn, does he look gray as a wolf in there.* He is not thriving. Luckily, I don't see shit on the floor, so that's a bonus.

I poke my head in and tell him I'm grabbing supplies and will be right in. He gives me a thumbs up, and I turn around to go to the clean room to grab everything I need. Again. As I'm grabbing my supplies, I'm wondering how in the world this man has anything left in his gut. It's not like he's eating anything. I guess that just goes to show you how much actual crap is built up in your system at any given time.

I go to grab a cloth Chux pad to put under him, and the entire pile falls onto the ground. MOTHER OF GOD. I go over to the counter and put down all the crap in my hands, then go pick it all up and restack them. Then I grab all my stuff again, and stand there with a blank stare, trying to make my brain work so I don't forget anything.

Okay, I'm pretty sure I have everything and start walking out the door.

As soon as I hear the door click behind me, I remember that I don't have any more wipes in Ron's room, so I badge back into the supply room and grab three packs because I can never be too prepared for this room.

Finally, I'm sure I'm good; I walk back out into the hallway and see Kirsten jogging down the hall with meds in her hands. As she passes me, I ask, "You good?"

"Yup, just intubating room 126," she replies over her shoulder.

Shit, I can't believe another one is getting intubated! Where in the hell are we going to put all these patients? Last I knew there was only one ICU bed open—and I'm praying for her patient that it's still open—but I wonder silently what will become of Ron. We will have to start using the ER if patients keep needing intubation.

I put all my supplies down on the table outside of Ron's room and start the lovely gowning process for the six thousandth time today. Turning on the lights, I ask Ron if he's okay and he answers, "I mean, this shit is getting old, ya know what I mean?"

Boy do I, buddy. I don't want to be cleaning you up any more than you want to be nonstop shitting yourself, trust me.

He knows the routine by now and lowers the head of his

bed while I get everything prepped. He has regained some of his strength, and with just a little help from me, he rolls onto his right side, and I start cleaning him up. I get the new linen all bunched up underneath him while carefully rolling the soiled ones onto themselves, making sure not to get poop on the clean ones.

(There is not much worse than having to do TWO bed changes because you weren't careful enough and got shit on your clean linens.)

I tug on his hip to indicate to him to turn onto his other side, and he doesn't respond like he usually does. I pull a bit harder and, as he rolls a little toward me, I see that he is foaming at the mouth.

He then starts convulsing with a full-blown seizure. I put him on his left side—in the "recovery position"—as best I can. I run to the door and yell out that I need Ativan for a seizure immediately, and Ryan gets up out of his chair and runs to the med room to override it without a doctor's order. We can only do this in emergency situations, and the docs put the order in afterward.

I go back to Ron and make sure that his head and neck are protected. I run the vitals machine, and see that his heart rate is 188, and his BP is 176/98. It's impossible to count his respiratory rate with all his movements, and I can't get a reliable heart rhythm reading either.

Thirty seconds later and he is still seizing. *Ugh.* I knew his gray coloring was bad news. He is moving around so much that the entire bed change I was doing is completely messed up, so that's awesome.

Ryan comes into the room gowned and gloved and hands me 4 mg of Ativan drawn up in a syringe. He tells me he told the docs, and they are on their way in. I immediately push the

Ativan and then flush his IV with saline when I'm done. A few seconds later, he stops seizing.

I take a deep breath and look at Ryan. He knows what I'm going to ask for and tells me he will be back with another bed change.

I watch him walk out the door and then glance down at Ron. He is covered in his own diarrhea again, and the foam is still all over his face. I grab a hand towel and wet it in the sink and carefully wipe his mouth and face off. His heart rate has come back down to 96, and I push the button to recycle the blood pressure reading. While it takes the measurement, I finish cleaning up his face and mouth and wipe his head off from the sweat with a cold cloth.

154/90. Better, but not awesome. He is not responsive. People in this "postictal" (after-seizure) state can take several minutes to several hours to get back to normal. Seizures are like making scrambled eggs out of your brain. Not good.

As I'm trying to get him to wake up and respond to me, the hospitalist doc and Ryan both come into the room. Ryan and I start cleaning him up, and the doc does a quick assessment and asks me what happened.

"It was a witnessed seizure of approximately 60 seconds in length, and it stopped with the administration of 4 mg of IV Ativan," I tell him, "He has no history of seizures."

The doc nods and says, "He hasn't been looking good all afternoon."

I totally agree as Ryan and I turn him once again and finalize the bed change and clean up. We prop him up in bed, incline the head of the bed slightly, and place his blankets back on top of him. He is starting to wake up a bit and starts moaning and grasping at his head.

Ron isn't really able to form words or communicate at this point. I stay at his bedside for another 15 minutes, fussing with his bedding, making sure he is clean, checking my handheld for new orders because I'm expecting them to start him on an antiseizure medication, like Keppra, at any moment. I organize and clean off his bedside table, then do the same for the area around his sink so there are clean workspaces and I can see what supplies I have in the room. My main reason for staying in here a while is to see if he has another seizure.

He doesn't seize again, and I see new med orders for him on my handheld, so I take off my garbage bag and head towards the med room. On my way, I'm told by the unit secretary that the PACU (Post Anesthesia Care Unit) nurse is on the line for me. She is waiting to give me report on Jerry's surgery, so I know what happened. I ask her to tell them that I'll call them back in a few minutes because I don't want to delay giving Ron his seizure meds.

I walk into the med room to get the meds and New Grad is standing in the middle of the room just staring into oblivion. I recognize her distant eyes. I put my hand gently on her shoulder, and she snaps out of it and looks at me, still reeling from her code earlier.

I ask her if she's doing okay, and she says she is. I tell her it's okay to not be okay, and she nods her head and walks out the door holding a cup full of meds.

Going over to the Pyxis machine, I open Ron's med profile and see that the Keppra hasn't been approved by pharmacy yet. I walk over to the phone and dial their extension. I ask the pharmacist who answers to please approve the med immediately so I can pull it from the Pyxis. She tells me she will do so right away, and I thank her and hang up. I imagine what it must be like to be a pharmacist right now in COVID times with a hospital full of super-sick people who need their meds ASAP all day and all night long. I wonder how many phone calls like that they get a day. I'd guess a hundred or more. *Yikes.*

5:20 PM

Standing in the med room scrolling through my handheld, I check out what I still have to get done on my shift for my other patients while I wait for her to approve the Keppra.

I suddenly remember that Jerry is down in PACU, pick up the phone again and call to get the report. I realize as I am listening to the ringing that I have nothing to write on, so I grab a wrinkly alcohol pad packet out of my pocket and get my pen ready.

Joanne, the PACU nurse, tells me that Jerry had severe diverticulitis and inflammation of his bowels. They did a colostomy and left his abdominal incision open and placed a wound VAC (Vacuum-Assisted Closure) in the incision, which promotes healing and prevents infection.

This means that he now has a colostomy bag. It also means that they were unable to close his incision—likely because of his size—so they had to leave it open and put a machine on it that applies suction to the area. This suction keeps the wound in a clean environment and starts the healing process until they can fully close the wound. Sometimes they can never surgically close it, so it has remain on until it heals as it is.

At this point, Joanne says, "He is a truly pleasant individual, isn't he?"

I respond, "OMG Jo, he is about the best patient I've ever had. Really, people like him are the reason I am in nursing, to be honest."

She laughs, tells me the drugs he was given during surgery and then tells me, "I'm sorry to report, but he is extubated and fully able to make his needs known."

I grumble at this but tell her I'm ready for him to come up whenever they need to get him out of there. We exchange goodbyes and hang up.

I put the three alcohol pads with my scribbles on them back into a different pocket, so I don't accidentally use them, and get Ron's meds out of the Pyxis. I see that he is also due for some nausea meds, so I get those out, on a hunch that he will have at least a little bit of that after the whole seizure rollercoaster.

I gown and glove back up and go into his room. He looks at me when I walk in, which I take as a good thing, but he still looks gray and sickly.

I explain to him which medications I have for him, and he slowly nods his head. I can't tell if much is sinking in. I do a full neurological exam, but don't find any noticeable deficits. He's still postictal and coming out of it slowly.

Ron takes his Keppra, and I give him his nausea meds via IV. He says thank you and sinks his head back into his pillow. I ask if he wants the TV on and he shakes his head no. I quietly degown, turn off his lights, and head back out into the hallway, closing the door gently behind me.

I look down the hallway and see them wheeling Jerry into his room already. Joy.

Heading into Jerry's room after gowning back up, I hear him laying into the post-surgical staff. He's complaining about the fact that he cannot eat solid food for the foreseeable future, and how cold it was down in the PACU. No one is really listening to him because I bet he's been doing this shit since they took the tube out of his throat down there.

We start talking over him, and they give me a quick bedside report, which is essentially a repeat of everything Joanne had already told me, and then they all leave.

I adjust his bed as low as it will go and organize and clean off his bedside table, ensuring his call light, phone, and all his precious gadgets are all in reach for him. I organize his sink area and empty the trashes because they are now overflowing. *The entire time* I am sorting out his room, this man is complaining.

He tells me the surgeons have no idea what they are doing because if they did, he wouldn't have this "stupid ostomy thing" and that, because of their inability to do their jobs correctly, he now has to shit into a bag.

I start trying to educate him about his surgery. Explaining to him the reason behind a colostomy, that it is almost always temporary, and that his guts need a rest. I have a lot more to explain to him, but he cuts me off so many times that I just shut up and listen to him complain.

He gets quiet for a minute, and I look over at him because this is not normal. I can tell he is tearing up and getting emotional. Walking over to his bed, I look him in the eyes. He touches his stomach and can feel the bag and the wound VAC and starts really crying now.

I hold onto his other hand, and he says, "I can't believe I'm going to shit into a bag. But I guess without this surgery . . . I could've ended up dead. . . ."

I just stand there, holding his hand, listening.

"I mean, I don't even know how I'm going to manage all of this! And the doctors said my stomach was left open? What does that even mean? When will they close it?"

He looks pleadingly into my eyes and I can tell that, this time, he actually wants me to tell him.

"Well," I say, taking a deep breath and sitting on the edge of his bed, "when someone has a surgery where they clean out a lot of infection, they often leave the incision line open. They do this so the tissues and organs in your abdomen have time to fight off any remaining infection, for the swelling to go down and for things to get back to normal. Sometimes they leave it for a couple of days, other times for a week or more. It depends how ill you are, how bad the infection is, and how well you are healing from the treatments and surgery."

He nods his head and asks, "Will I have a harder time healing because of how big I am?"

Still holding his hand, I make eye contact and tell him, "Yes, it can mean healing takes longer and it also means you are more at risk for side effects and complications than someone of a normal weight. The main one is going to be incision healing. When they are finally able to close you up in a few days, unfortunately there's a high risk that the incision line will open back up on its own."

He says okay, and I can tell this session is over. I stand up and let go of his hand. As I push his bedside table back toward him, he starts back in on me, "Where are my applesauces and chips that were on my table before I left?"

I stare at him in awe for a second because we literally just got done talking about how his obesity is causing him life-threatening issues, and he knows that he can't have any food any time soon. It's clear he has no ability to truly comprehend the severity of his morbid obesity. This is a true food addiction.

I explain, "I threw them away because they were days old, and you are not going to be eating solid food for several days."

He starts calling me names, telling me I'm stupid, and that if I had any sense in my brain, I would have set them aside for the future. I just start ripping off my garbage bag and walk out of the room mid-sentence.

Again.

I stand in the hallway and look at the time. *It's fricking 5:45 pm.* I have one hour to get all my shit done, plus documentation.

I walk to Barb's room and poke my head in the door. "Hey Barb, how are you feeling, do you need more pain meds?"

"Yes, please," she says as loudly as she can over her BiPAP machine.

I go to the med room and grab her morphine and Ativan,

and go back to her room and get garbage-bag beautiful before heading in. Feeling guilty about how little I've been in her room, I get to her bedside and she immediately asks me when she can get home. I tell her we are waiting on confirmation of hospital bed delivery, and she nods understandingly. As I give her the IV medications, I watch her close her eyes and fold her hands on her stomach, waiting patiently to get home where she will be surrounded by love and comfort.

I think how desperate I would be if I were her to get home as I take my garbage bag off and walk out of the room. I stand in the hallway rubbing the hand sanitizer into my hands, thinking how precious the ability to die at home, surrounded by loved ones and a familiar scene, is for me.

In my opinion, dying in a hospital is a terrible way to go, and it's such a shame that so many hundreds of thousands of people have to do it, without even being given an honest choice or chance to have it any other way.

I walk by Tim's room and see on the monitor that he is still (oxygen) saturating in the 90s without BiPAP on. *FINALLY, a success story.* For now. It's common for people being weaned off BiPAP to then get a cytokine storm that fills their lungs back up with a bunch of fluid and infection, and they are put back on BiPAP or emergently intubated, depending on the severity. I pray this is not the case for him.

I also see there is more urine in his urinal, and almost cry a happy tear. After donning my PPE, I head in and tell him again how proud I am of him using his urinal correctly. He smiles big and asks if he can have something to eat. I message the doc to ask if we can get a diet order in for him and tell Tim I'll get him something once this goes through.

I am so happy to see this right now. Patting him on the shoulder, I take my gear back off and walk out.

I notice that room 112's call light is on, so I head down to see Roxy, who is clearly short of breath. I put my gear on as quickly as possible and head into her room. As I'm closing the door behind me, she looks up with panic in her eyes, just like she did this morning when her sugar tanked.

As soon as I've hooked her up to the vitals machine, I grab the glucometer and check her sugar. *Glucose of 380,* so that is slowly improving. But her oxygen is only 82%, so I put her on 4L nasal canula—four liters per minute of oxygen through a nose tube. After a few minutes, she only goes up to 84%, so I crank it up to 10L.

This only gets her up to 88%, so I call respiratory therapy (RT) and ask them to bring a BiPAP machine to her room. They tell me they are on their way, so I hang up and then call the doc and ask them to come into the room because she is decompensating (her lungs aren't working well enough despite the increase in oxygen therapy).

While I'm waiting, I increase her oxygen to 15L, and she is barely hitting 90%. My phone rings and I answer it. It's RT. There are no more BiPAPs in-house. *Word.*

I press the call button and ask for a high-flow nasal canula and an over-the-nose-and-mouth oxygen mask. The unit secretary brings them to me, so I hook Roxy up to 10L via high-flow nasal canula and then put 15L via oxygen mask on top of that.

Okay, I got her up to 93%. *Finally.* I take a deep breath of relief.

The doc pokes his head in the door and asks what happened. I tell him that I think her lungs are starting to give out because of the COVID, and that she needs to be on BiPAP, but that there are no available BiPAP machines in-house. I tell him the oxygen I have her on, and he sighs and says, "Okay, we will keep a close eye on her."

Roxy's eyes are again full of fear, but she is less short of breath than when I came first into the room. I tell her that it will be okay, and that it's important that she stays calm and relaxed to allow her lungs to work the best they can. I suggest that if she can tolerate it, she should lay on her stomach to increase the expansion of her lungs, and she nods her head. I make sure she is all tucked in, empty her trashes, degown, and head into the hallway.

On my way to the dirty linen room with several garbage bags, I see Kirsten walking past room 113, Ron's room. She yells "Tiff! Ron doesn't look too good in there...."

I chuck the garbage bags into the bin and run down the hall. *Why didn't I look in his window when I passed his room?! What was I thinking?*

I grab a gown, look in the window, and can tell he is not currently breathing.

FUCK BALLS.

I don't even tie my gown; I run into his room and check for a pulse. Nothing. I slam the code blue button on the wall, get the bed into CPR position, and immediately start compressions. I can hear the loud-ass code cart being wheeled this way, and Kirsten comes to the door with it, gowned up already.

6:00 PM

Kirsten immediately starts pulling open the drawers and says "17:58 CPR start time" as she scribbles this down on a piece of scrap paper. She grabs her phone and starts a timer, and we start the two-minute cycle count for each round.

People start flooding into the room. The doc immediately starts calling the shots and assigns roles to people—Emma is pushing drugs; Kirsten is the scribe. The pharmacist Shawn comes to the doorway and starts opening all the drawers just outside the room and drawing up medications to hand over to Emma. She has to open the door to hand the meds through for each request. Ryan is behind me telling me he will do compressions once my two minutes is up, and a panel of docs are standing there trying to figure out the cause of this cardiac arrest.

Two minutes goes by, we do a pulse check; have nothing on the monitor and no palpable pulse, so Ryan continues compressions as epinephrine is pushed quickly. It has been found that pushing epinephrine while doing chest compressions significantly increases the circulation of the drug, which makes sense if you think about how the heart works.

I get the CPR board from the code cart, and New Grad and I get it positioned, as well as the back automated external defibrillator (AED) pad read because once the next two-minute check comes up, we will turn him onto his side, place the AED pad on his left shoulder blade, and slide the board underneath him.

Ryan is starting to sweat because it's hot AF in these rooms with all these people and all this stupid gear.

Two-minute check again—we place the board and put the pad on and get him back supine ASAP to do a true pulse check. No pulse, asystole. No epinephrine this round, but doc orders sodium bicarbonate to attempt to keep his pH as normal as possible. Blood gets acidic because of lactic acid and carbon dioxide retention and the effects of the epinephrine; the sodium bicarbonate will not normalize it but will hopefully stop it getting too far out of whack, which is very dangerous.

I start compressions again, which is fine by me. I prefer doing compressions over any other position on the code team. First of all, I use it as a core exercise (don't judge me). Also, it's relatively brainless. I literally just sing "Stayin' Alive" by the Bee Gees in my head to stay on beat (at just over 100 beats per minute, the song is the right tempo for CPR compressions), and don't have to think about much else.

We go through five rounds of this, and at ten minutes, we still have no pulse. This means that Ron has been effectively dead for ten minutes. It's possible to get him back, but he will likely never be "normal" again. Usually, after this long, patients have what's called an anoxic brain injury, meaning their brain tissue has died or is dying from not having enough oxygen.

On round six, Ryan is doing compressions, and I change out my gloves because sweat is literally coming out of them when I do my compressions. During pulse check, they find a weak pulse, and the monitor says HR 130, but it's V-tach (ventricular tachycardia): the heart's ventricles are beating too fast and contracting out of control. So, we shock with AED and then don't have a pulse again.

I restart compressions, and the docs decide to intubate.

The airway cart is being pulled down the hallway, and supplies are being handed into the room like a chain of workers on the railway. They move the bed down away from the wall a bit so the docs can fit at the head of the bed.

It's a real treat to keep doing effective compressions with a moving target underneath you, let me tell you. My forearms are starting to get tired, but I think in my brain that this is just a workout, and I can handle anything.

I see the ventilator machine being wheeled in and hooked up by RT out of the corner of my eye. They prep him for intubation, and at the next pulse check, he is pulseless and intubated without sedation because he is not alive. We start compressions again once the tube is in, and he is bagged via the life support tube with an Ambu-bag. Ryan does his compressions while I clean up a tad, trying to make the area more workable.

Next pulse check, we get a pulse at 140, sinus tachycardia, which means his heart is still going too fast, but the rhythm is survivable. We stop compressions, hook him up to the ventilator, and I can hear the doc on the phone with the ICU. They say that the room we had our eyes on from earlier is almost cleaned so he can likely go down soon.

Apparently, Kirsten's patient must have died, and I immediately feel bad that I didn't help or ask her about it.

In the meantime, the code team all stay in the room because the chances of him coding again are very high. If the ICU room doesn't get clean in the next ten minutes or so, Ron will have to go down into the ER for holding until an ICU bed opens because we cannot keep intubated people on the medical floor.

We all start to organize things, talk through the code to see if there was anything we should have done better or differently. We come up with no process improvements, except that maybe he should have been on continuous monitoring. The problem with that on our floor is that we don't have any central monitors. For example, in the ICU, they have several stations where there are monitors showing everyone's continuously monitored vital signs, heart rhythms, and especially oxygenation status. If someone starts tanking or coding up there, they know within seconds.

Here on the floor, even if I had him on continuous monitoring, it would have to register in the telemetry room, and they would then have to call me on my phone to tell me that something was weird in one of my rooms.

Often, alarms go off not due to a real rhythm issue, but because the patient is coughing, scratching, or just shifting in bed. These false alarms waste precious minutes and seconds in the coding world but are unavoidable on most med-surg units across the nation, as they have less sophisticated monitoring equipment than the ICU. Having centralized monitoring is expensive and labor intensive, and technically if a patient is on the med-surg floor they should (in most cases) be healthy enough to NOT need continuous monitoring.

So, if that is our only process improvement for this code, then we are doing well. I'm cleaning up his bed, under his bed, around his bed, and making sure all the equipment now attached to him is functioning and doesn't need to be adjusted. He's at 100% oxygen on the vent, and I see that his saturation is 100%, so I titrate the oxygen down to 80% to see where that holds him. Some coworkers are helping, but some go back to their rooms because we are all busy and it's coming up to the end of shift.

As he is intubated, we can't leave Ron alone in the room. So, if they can't bring him up to the ICU right away, I will have to ask for some help. Pre-COVID, there was always an ICU bed open for this type of shitshow, and I would have done a rapid response when he seized, and he would have likely been brought up to the ICU right then. But now, in these glorious times we are living in, patients are only brought up to the ICU if there is an open bed and if they are intubated.

Open ICU beds are like gold nowadays.

I do a neuro check on him to see where he is at because he is not currently sedated, which means he should be VERY uncomfortable; he has a breathing tube, and we just pounded on his chest for over a quarter of an hour.

Unfortunately, Ron's pupils are blown with no reflexivity; he has no gag reflex when I suction his tube; he has no reaction to painful stimuli; and has no corneal reflex when I check it as a last resort.

Not good.

Usually, absence of all reflexes is highly indicative of a full anoxic brain injury or brain death. *Shit, I hope this isn't true . . .* but it's not looking good.

I hear Ryan get a phone call from the ICU saying that the room is ready, so we immediately start wheeling him up there. The charge nurse from up there was already down on the floor and walks up with us. Once we get to the room, I give my report to the primary nurse.

I make sure the ICU nurses don't need anything from me after we transfer him into their critical care bed and report is done. They all have empty eyes like I have never seen before . . .

I can't imagine what they are going through up there, I really can't. Their patients are sick as shit, they never get a break, they are fucked all day every day. . . .

Actually, so are we.

I degown and hand Ron's chart to their unit secretary with a weary smile that she can't even see because of my dumb mask. A sudden wave of extreme exhaustion washes over me as I head back down to my floor. It's 6:42 pm.

6:45 PM

I get back down to the floor, and I see an ambulance crew outside of room 111, Barb's room. *Hallelujah!* They must have gotten confirmation and arranged transport while I was dealing with Ron.

I get a tear in my eye, probably because I am so overtired and burnt out, but also because I am so happy that she lived long enough to go home to die in the way that she wants to. My shoulders ache as I gown and glove and head into the room where the ambulance crew is doing their initial assessment and gathering her belongings.

While helping them, I give a quick report as they hook her up to their oxygen to make sure she will get home alive. Once she is all bundled up and ready to go, I hold her hand and look in her eyes and tell her I wish her luck and peace and comfort.

She has a tear in her eye as she squeezes my hand, and they wheel her off.

I tidy up her room a bit because they will come and clean it and it will be filled again within the hour. I empty the trashes and linen cart, degown, and bring it all to the dirty utility room. This room smells so bad, I can't handle it, even with my N95 on. I get out as quick as possible and stand in the hallway for a second.

I have another moment, like so many before, where I stand with a blank, "stroking out" look on my face.

Melanie, the night shift nurse taking over my patients, comes up to me and puts a hand on my arm, snapping me out of my hazy fog.

"Oh hey," I say exhaustedly.

"Hey hun, just give me the down and dirty on your remaining people, I'm sure you've had a hell of a day from the rumors around here."

My remaining patients. *Remaining.* I had seven, down to four. Only one of whom is truly BETTER than when I started four days ago. One definitively dead. One basically dead. One going home to die. One going down the tubes toward death, one not getting better or worse, and one at very high risk of going down the shitter.

Jesus, what a crew. What a week. Honestly, I can't believe I didn't have at least one admission this shift. I'm pretty sure Ryan was taking it easy on me. I smile weakly, but it doesn't reach my eyes, so I'm sure she can't even tell.

We head over to my little corner computer area, and I tell her about the ever-pleasant Jerry, Roxy and her crazy sugars, Mildred and her pending surgery, and Tim—my only success story. She can't BELIEVE he finally pissed in a urinal. Basically, the whole floor is happy about it because, damn, what a pain in all our asses that was.

Melanie and I give each other a quick hug—we are kind of like each other's spirit animals . . . we have very similar personalities and souls. Thank GOD she was the night shift nurse relieving me tonight.

It's 6:58 pm. I still have an enormous amount of charting to do, so I turn to my computer and power it on as I apologize in advance to Melanie for anything I missed or overlooked or didn't have time to do. She waves me off, just like I would do to her, and gets to work.

First, I do my report on Ron's code. I do my documentation on Tim's incredible improvement (he ate 100% of the dinner that Dee graciously ordered for him during my shitshow in room 113). I make sure all of Roxy's blood sugars have transferred over and notice that one of the other nurses gave her her evening dose of insulin.

What would I do without my amazing coworkers? We each hold each other up with utmost respect, even if we don't hang out outside of work. None of us would be able to do this job (at least not well) without a team like this. I say a little prayer of gratitude and finish documenting on her day.

Then I head to Jerry's chart, record everything that happened there, and say another littler prayer of thanks that I never had to go back into that room again. I saw a glimpse of his humanity there, but it does not excuse the *literal abuse* that he puts us all through.

Next, I make sure everything is charted and complete in poor Juan's chart, and make sure to document the conversation with his family, and where his body and personal belongings ended up.

I finish up Barb's chart, making sure that all orders and instructions are where they should be because her hospice company will need all that information. Finally comes Mildred's chart, and I make sure the photos that were taken earlier of her foot are properly uploaded. *That feels like a different day, it was so long ago.* . . .

Rubbing my eyes and stretching back in my chair, I look at the time. 8:12 pm. *Shit!* My twelve-hour shift has almost turned into 14 hours.

I log out of the computer, gather my belongings (including my coffee cup that still has coffee in it), and go to the break room. I put all my stay-at-work crap in my locker and mindlessly pack everything else up to take home with me. I don't take my N95 mask off quite yet because I still have to walk some of the halls to get out of this place.

Putting my coat on, I make sure I have everything and head out the door. As I'm walking toward the stairs, I hear a call light going off, and a shout for help down the hallway. It takes everything in me not to respond to that, but I keep walking and close the door to the stairwell behind me.

I head down the stairs to the entrance to the parking garage and keep telling myself not to break down until I get to my car. I swipe my badge to clock out and heave a sigh of relief.

8:30 PM

I find my car, unlock it, throw my bag in the back, and get in the driver's seat. Starting it up, I literally RIP my N95 off my face. I take the little foam pad off my nose and look at it in my rearview mirror. No major breakdown today, thank God. I accidentally make eye contact with myself and then I lose it.

Covering my face with my hands, I just sob. My body wracks with grief, exhaustion, and relief that it is over for a few days.

Did I do enough? How could I have saved Juan or Ron? Could I have prevented Barbara's death?

All these questions feel legit in my heart. But rationally, I know there is nothing I could have done.

The sense of desperate inferiority and ineffectiveness that

takes over after a shift like this sometimes feels like too much to handle.

My brain feels so full and yet so empty at the same time. I pull myself together a tad, wipe my eyes, and put my car in reverse.

I get home safely, but don't remember a single thing about the drive. I do know that I had no music or anything on because my brain could not handle the stimulation. Parking my car in the driveway, I sit there for another moment in silence. I have to go into that house and leave all of this behind, or at least as much as I can.

I cannot let my kids see the amount of suffering in my eyes and laying heavy on my soul.

I hype myself up, turn off the car, and head to the door.

I take off my shoes outside and as I open the door, I can smell dinner. Suddenly I'm *starving*. I feel like I didn't eat at all today, which is basically true.

My kids come running to the door and, although I want to hug them so badly, I tell them to wait until after I shower, but that I love them and can't wait to snuggle on them. I yell to my husband that I love him and am going to shower. He says he loves me too, and I walk up the stairs.

I slowly peel off my gross contaminated scrubs. I put them in the plastic bag I have designated for our COVID clothes (since he works in the ICU with COVID patients all the time too). When I do work laundry, I use extra-hot settings and extra rinses. I double- and triple-check that none of the kids' belongings get anywhere near it.

Turning on the shower, I stand there while it heats up like a weird dog waiting for a treat. I am so excited about this hot shower; I couldn't begin to tell you. Once it's steaming, I get in the tub under the water and soon my entire body begins to release. I do some deep breathing and begin to cry again.

This is my favorite place to cry out my lingering emotions. Private, quiet, but also the water is loud enough that no one can hear me. I kneel on the floor of the tub, curl into the fetal position, and just sob.

I sob huge, gut-wrenching sobs of grief. I can feel snot coming out of my nose, but I don't care. I haven't done this in months, and hundreds of hours of built-up feelings of helplessness, frustration, and anger are all coming out at once.

I stay curled on the floor of the tub for at least five minutes, letting it out. Because, if I don't do this, it all stays in there like a toxin.

Once I finally stop crying, I stand back up and clean myself. Showering with purpose and gratitude, I am thankful that I am in my house; in my hot shower; with my healthy and happy family downstairs waiting for me.

If there is anything that COVID has taught me, it is to appreciate life to its fullest every single day.

I get out of the shower—only because you can't stay in there forever, unfortunately—and I dry off and get in some comfy clothes. As I walk down the stairs, the kids run to the bottom to greet me. I give them the hugest hug ever. God, I love their smell and their tiny bodies. They already ate dinner and are all ready for bed, but they sit at the table with me as I eat my dinner.

Behind the kids' backs, my husband holds up a bottle of wine in his right hand, and a bottle of vodka in his left hand with a questioning glance my way. I point towards his left hand, and he makes me my favorite drink (a vodka cranberry) and brings it to me.

He kisses my head, rubs my shoulders for a second, and asks what he can do for me. My brain is fried, but I really don't need anything, so that's what I tell him. I am just so grateful for this food and my kids being well taken care of.

Once I'm done eating, I clean up my dishes and head upstairs with the kids to their rooms.

I start the tuck-in and goodnight process with my youngest. He is six, and understands that COVID is bad, and can make you sick, and that I work with people that have it every day. He asks how my day was, and I tell him it was pretty rough. I tell him I had very sick patients, and a couple of them didn't make it. He puts his tiny hand on my arm in silence. It's like he knows there are no words for this shitshow. We read a book, I kiss him goodnight and tell him to have sweet dreams and that I'll see him in the morning.

Next, I head to my older son's room. He is nine and is watching videos on his phone. I tell him to put it away, and he does. I rub his back a bit, give him a little face massage, and ask about his day. He got a 100% on his spelling test that he is super proud of but says that he hates going to school remotely. He then asks how my day was, and I repeat what I said to his brother. He also just lays there silently, knowing no words really work here, but eventually whispers, "Those people are lucky that you and other nurses are there."

I think about this for a sec and realize that he is totally right. Without nurses, what would the world be doing right now? I thank him and give him a kiss and hug and say goodnight.

I go back downstairs to my husband sitting on the couch with one of our playlists going on the stereo in the background. He has my drink, refilled, sitting on a coaster on the table.

He raises his head when he hears me walking into the room and I sit down next to him, heavily. He pulls me into his chest and gently strokes my hair even though it's still damp. He asks me no questions. He knows.

It's so nice to be with someone who truly *knows*. We sit there and sip on our drinks until they are gone, and I start to drift in and out of consciousness. Usually, I would stay up and drink a little more, or at least start a movie, but after today, and after four days like this in a row, I just absolutely can't do it. I get up, put my glass in the sink, and head back upstairs.

I brush my teeth and do my quick skin care routine, all the while trying not to make eye contact with myself in the mirror. I make sure everything is charging and in its right place and lay into bed.

Oh. My. God. These clean, cold, delicious-smelling sheets are the best place on this earth, I promise you.

My feet are absolutely pounding, and I can feel the circulation trying to be restored down there. The alcohol has quieted my brain a little but not a ton. I snuggle deeply into my man's chest, breathing heavily and purposefully.

Eventually, I drift off to sleep, safe from the tormenting nightmares of work.

Mostly.

PART TWO

THE RUDDERLESS SHIP

FROM ONE SHIFT TO THE WHOLE DAMN SYSTEM

What you have just read is a sample of a real shift as a registered nurse (RN) in America during the pandemic. It wasn't written dramatized for effect, it's what it was—one day, one nurse.

I wish I could say it was the worst of them—but it wasn't. Days like that happened all the time during the pandemic. And honestly, they still happen now.

What I experienced in those twelve hours was not just the emotional weight of death, chaos, and exhaustion, it was the direct result of a broken system. A system that underpays, overworks, and dehumanizes its workers. A system that lets patients slip through the cracks because administrators are too busy counting dollars to count safe staffing ratios. A system where band-aids are sold at markup while lives unravel.

What you read was the symptom. What comes next is the diagnosis.

Because it's not just about burnout. It's about greed. Bureaucracy. Corporate medicine. Insurance companies making life-or-death decisions. Pharmaceutical giants manipulating the market. Politicians too far removed from hospital beds to care.

If you're angry, good. If you're heartbroken, even better. This means you're paying attention. Because this isn't just my story—it's the story of every healthcare worker and patient trapped in this system.

Now let's pull the curtain all the way back and talk about what's *really* going on.

CHAPTER 1

FEAR AND RESILIENCE
CONFRONTING COVID'S UNSEEN IMPACT

WE ARE at a pivotal moment in the history of healthcare, both in America and across the globe. The aftermath of a global pandemic has left its mark on all of us, particularly those of us in the trenches of healthcare. COVID-19 swept into our lives with little warning—sudden, ferocious, and entirely disruptive. As a nurse with 15 years of experience, I've worked across many different areas of nursing, and I was in the thick of it throughout this crap. Like so many in my field, I experienced a whirlwind of emotions during the crisis.

At the start of the pandemic, I was fueled by a fiery determination to rise to the occasion. I felt a profound sense of purpose—to save lives, to confront the unknown, and to work under conditions that many might consider unthinkable. At one point, I even registered with a travel-nurse agency, eager to go to New York City, where the crisis was the worst, to help those who needed care the most. (Pro tip: if you're a nurse, don't sign up with a travel agency unless you're truly ready to commit—take my word for it.)

I wanted to be the hero that the media, administrators, and government officials were praising nurses to be.

In those early days, my morale soared. I felt vital—my skills, my knowledge, and my training felt like they were not just valuable but critical to the survival of my community and even the world. Signs appeared in front of hospitals, proclaiming healthcare workers as heroes. I felt an unshakable camaraderie with my colleagues. We were united by purpose, bonded by a collective mission to confront an unprecedented challenge. I even posted on social media, trying to calm the anxiety that seemed to overwhelm everyone around me. Family, friends, and neighbors were in a state of near panic, and even many healthcare workers were rattled, afraid of what we might face.

Some of my coworkers refused to take care of COVID-positive patients. Others left the profession altogether, unable to come to terms with the risks to their personal lives. It was a tumultuous time, but I never doubted my role.

Those closest to me were terrified for my safety, but I carried an unwavering belief that I was where I needed to be, doing what I was meant to do. My dad even sent me a box of 1,000 ponchos to use as makeshift PPE in case the hospital ran out of gowns—a precaution that, shockingly, wasn't as absurd as it sounds.

Through it all, I was not afraid. Not once did I fear COVID—not for a single moment. I believed that if the universe had decided I was going to get COVID and die from it, there was nothing I could do to prevent that outcome. It's a way of thinking that some might find unsettling, but for me, it brought clarity and focus. My mom taught me to never fear dying, but to expect and respect it. That lesson stayed with me through every shift, and every interaction with a COVID-positive patient.

To this day, I haven't gotten COVID, and I don't believe I ever will.

Of course, it wasn't all smooth sailing. There were moments of frustration and exhaustion, especially during the early days. Working as an ER nurse in a small community hospital at the time, I was frustrated by the lack of PPE, the constantly shifting guidelines, and the endless deluge of conflicting information. The science was evolving by the hour, and it was infuriating to try to keep up, while also reassuring patients who were understandably terrified.

As I watched my coworkers, I saw them dismiss their real experiences and just blindly believe the media rhetoric. I would ask questions about things that were changes from the norm, or that didn't make sense to me, and I was dismissed and told to get in line.

I got real tired of explaining to people that a positive test or even severe symptoms didn't necessarily mean a death sentence. I grew equally tired of the stigma attached to healthcare workers. Walking into a grocery store or public space in scrubs felt like walking around with a scarlet letter (I do this very rarely, but ya know... kids).

People stared, some even recoiled, as if I were a walking disease. It was isolating and disheartening, especially in a small town where everyone knew one another.

But maybe what bothered me most was the fear—the pervasive, overwhelming fear that seemed to take hold of everyone. The media played a significant role in fueling that fear, bombarding people with headlines and stories that often did more harm than good. While it's true that COVID was a serious illness, the media seemed to only focus on worst-case scenarios, and it created a level of anxiety that was debilitating for many.

There's a clip of a news reporter from about a year into the pandemic, admitting he was tired of reporting on COVID every single day. *I bet you were tired, bro!* We were all tired. Tired of the fear, the misinformation, and the relentless constant focus on doom and gloom.

The reality—as I saw it from the front lines—was far more nuanced than the media portrayed.

Yes, COVID was serious, and yes, it claimed many lives. But the narrative of inevitable death for anyone who contracted the virus was simply not real. For most people, the risk of severe outcomes was low, yet the fear persisted, fueled by endless media coverage and speculation from uneducated officials.

As healthcare workers, we bore most of the weight of that fear—not just our own, but the fear of our patients, their families, and our communities. It was exhausting, both emotionally and physically. Yet through it all, I kept coming back to the same belief: I was exactly where I needed to be. I didn't have all the answers, and I certainly didn't always feel like a hero, but I felt like my work mattered.

Now that we are at the end of this debacle, I find myself reflecting on what we've learned—and what we've yet to address. The pandemic exposed cracks in our healthcare system, in our leadership, and our overall resources as a country and world. It forced us to confront uncomfortable truths about fear, misinformation, and the human tendency to catastrophize.

According to the *New York Times* in May 2022, approximately 82 million Americans had tested positive for COVID-19 since the start of the pandemic.[1] (It's important to note that this figure includes an unknown number of false-positive results, and likely false-negatives too.) During the same period, according to the *Wall Street Journal*, the reported death toll was 997,001.[2] When you put these figures together, the resulting mortality rate was 1.2% among those who contracted the virus —not the total population of the United States.

If you have lost someone you love to COVID, my heart goes out to you. Every life lost is a tragedy, and these deaths were deeply painful for the individuals, families, and communities affected. Each person mattered, and their absence is felt.

However, when we examine the data objectively, the vast majority of those who died were individuals with preexisting conditions, obesity, or advanced age—factors that placed them in high-risk categories for severe outcomes from COVID or similar illnesses.

The deaths caused by COVID-19 are no laughing matter. It's a reminder of the virus' devastating impact, especially on vulnerable populations. But alongside the grief and reflection, we need to acknowledge the unnecessary fear that was—and continues to be—instilled in the general public. The level of fear promoted by media coverage, while understandable early on due to the unknowns surrounding the virus, became excessive and created widespread anxiety that still exists today.

To provide some perspective, consider the mortality rate of smallpox, a disease that once ravaged through populations. Historical data suggests that smallpox killed between 20% and 45% of those it infected.[3] COVID's mortality rate of 1.2% (based on reported cases) pales in comparison. Of course, modern medical advancements and public health measures play a critical role in reducing mortality from infectious diseases, but even without these factors, smallpox was far more lethal.

Again, this is not to diminish the seriousness of COVID, but to emphasize the context.

Smallpox was so deadly that its outbreaks were catastrophic on a scale modern society can hardly fathom. A disease with a mortality rate upwards of 20% would overwhelm healthcare systems and devastate populations in ways we can't even imagine today. COVID, while dangerous and tragic in its own right, does not begin to compare to that level of lethality.

The Spanish Flu pandemic of 1918 is estimated to have claimed the lives of 50 million people worldwide over the course of just two years.[4] In comparison, as of October 2024, COVID is estimated to have caused approximately seven million deaths globally.[5] These numbers paint a stark contrast and provide an opportunity for reflection and perspective.

Let me be even more clear: I have seen firsthand the devastation this virus caused. I've witnessed patients endure unimaginable suffering, and I know how deeply this disease has affected many lives. However, it is equally important to step back and examine the broader picture. The portrayal of COVID's impact by the media often took public fear to extreme levels. The resulting mental health crisis, increased suicide rates, riots, and panic-driven behaviors—such as hoarding essential supplies—created life-threatening challenges of their own.

Take, for example, the coverage of Italy in the early months of the pandemic, particularly around May 2020. Images and videos of overwhelmed hospitals and mass casualties dominated headlines, creating an atmosphere of panic and despair worldwide. While Italy, like much of the world, did have a difficult time with COVID, it has since been revealed that much of the footage was repeatedly recycled and may not have reflected the full reality on the ground. According to data, Italy's overall death rate during the pandemic was 0.73%—less than 1%.[6]

This is not to downplay the severity of the situation in Italy, but it does highlight how the media's focus, exaggerations and lies contributed to an unneeded level of fear.

As the primary wound care provider in my hospital's COVID ICU during the height of the pandemic, I witnessed the daily impact of COVID. I saw patients deteriorate so quickly, progressing from shortness of breath to reliance on continuous BiPAP machines (which help force air into the lungs to improve breathing), and eventually to intubation. Once intubated, many of these patients' spent weeks on life support. For some, there was no improvement, and they were transitioned to palliative care, either passing away in the hospital or, if they were fortunate, at home surrounded by loved ones.

Others underwent tracheostomies—a surgical procedure that creates an opening in the neck for a plastic tube to maintain an open airway. For those who survived, many required long-term care, remaining dependent on machines for the rest of their lives. Only a handful were able to have their tracheostomies reversed and return to a semblance of normalcy.

I remember looking younger patients in the eye, having conversations with them, and then hearing just a few days later that they had passed away. I watched the unrelenting toll this took on my colleagues. ICU nurses, day after day, made phone calls to families with little to no good news to share. Many of them endured weeks where every single patient they cared for died. I saw the exhaustion and numbness in their eyes—a weariness that no amount of sleep could fix.

For new nurses who graduated in May 2020, their first experiences in the field were nothing short of insanity. They entered the profession during an unprecedented crisis and were immediately put into the chaos of a global pandemic. Many of them were in a state of shock, grappling with the harsh realities of a career they had only just started.

I came up to the unit one day, and my coworker told me that 15 people had died on our 20-bed unit in the last 36 hours. That's an average of a death every two hours.

This pandemic has taken more from us than just the lives of patients. Nurses will lose our own for years to come because of this. Not just from the increased depression, suicide, and burnout, but because this has taken the souls and brains and hearts from healthcare workers across the globe. The stress and strain of living in sorrow and pain for years will not go without consequences.

And then there's this weird "warzone state" where we were all under this intense pressure and felt like we were making an enormous difference in the world. We were desperately needed, and we were saving lives. In those chaotic days, breaks were a luxury we couldn't afford and, some days, we couldn't even leave the unit.

In the ICU, we spent hours in the rooms of critically ill patients, managing endless crises. The action never stopped. You'd leave one room only to run into another to start chest compressions. The pace was relentless, and as awful as it is to admit, many of us became accustomed to the adrenaline. Now that intensity has died down, some of us feel strangely out of place. There's a pervasive sense of guilt because that "action" was fueled by human suffering and death.

How do we reconcile feeling unfulfilled in a time of relative calm? How do we process emotions so difficult to explain?

One of the most difficult events to witness and participate in is the death of one person, only to then immediately move on to continue to care for more dying people. I describe in Part I how New Grad experiences her first death; something that thousands of healthcare workers experience every day. The emotional toll it takes to watch life leave someone's eyes, to then have to tell their loved ones about it, and then immediately have to move on as if nothing has happened is honestly crazy. And there was a different level to it during the pandemic because so few people were improving. Obviously, it is horrible to lose a loved one . . . but to lose patient after patient is something that's very difficult to describe unless you were there.

Recently, I tried reading a book written by a fellow

COVID ICU nurse, *Year of the Nurse: A Covid-19 2020 Pandemic Memoir*.[7] I hoped it would provide a fresh perspective and give me insight into another healthcare worker's experience. Instead, I found page after page of political blame, anger, and divisiveness. Rather than offering a reflective memoir or an informative exploration of the crisis, the book was filled with vitriol.

The author shared how she relied on medications like Ativan and Ambien to cope and made it clear that she resented anyone who didn't share her political views. She literally starts her book with, "If you mind-bogglingly voted for Trump, please stop reading and go ask for a refund." Throughout the book, she stands on a podium of superiority, lecturing her family constantly, and even going as far as wishing Republicans dead.

This kind of rhetoric was deeply upsetting to me. Every healthcare professional, regardless of political beliefs, suffered during the pandemic. We all showed up, we all did the work, and we all carried the weight of the lives lost. This author's hatred and anger felt like a betrayal of the shared experience we all endured. The pandemic didn't discriminate by political party, nor did the suffering it caused. Nurses, whether conservative, liberal, or apolitical, worked side by side often at the expense of our mental and physical health.

We all chose this profession. We knew the responsibility it carried, and we embraced the challenges it brought. Those who couldn't handle the demands of nursing during the pandemic made the understandable and respectable decision to leave. But to weaponize the profession, to blame entire groups of people for suffering, is shameful and dishonors the sacrifice we all made.

In a way, TV shows like *Grey's Anatomy*, *Superstore*, and *South Park* glorified the pandemic. *Grey's Anatomy* has been my favorite TV show since before I was even I nurse. Most of how they portrayed the pandemic was pretty real . . . especially in the beginning when we knew very little about the disease. But they took it much too far in many instances, and that made what we were going through on the real front lines seem not as intense or important.

Yes, we had to quarantine, but very, very few healthcare workers chose to not go home for weeks on end because they were treating COVID patients. Proper precautions were taken, but we still went home. Exhausted and defeated, we *needed* to go home more than anything.

There's a difference between the fear of a healthcare worker bringing home COVID to her children after treating positive, dying patients all day, and the fear of someone going into a grocery store. These shows and the media depicted a world that made these two fears equal, and that's bullshit.

Walking into your own home and not touching anything or anyone until you take a shower (while leaving your shoes outside and bagging your scrubs separately from all other clothes) is an experience that is very difficult to describe. Having to teach your kids that they can't hug or touch you when you get home from a 13-hour shift adds to the depression, sadness, and mental exhaustion. That is NOT the same as being scared of contracting COVID while you decide between Apple Jacks and Cheerios.

Let me illustrate the destructive power of fear with a case history.

I had a patient in the ER: a 16-year-old girl who came directly from school because she was having a full-blown panic attack and could hardly breathe. She was so scared of getting COVID and dying that she could not mentally handle it. She lost hours at school, kids were making fun of her, and she struggled for the rest of the year with anxiety and depression.

She was completely terrified and shaking when she came

into the ER. I sat on the side of her bed and tried to explain that even if she did get COVID, the chances of her getting super sick—and especially of dying—were so small that they almost didn't exist.

Because of the media, she didn't believe me.

Yeah, I got sick of that shit pretty quick.

But generally, the anxiety the public felt and feels about being exposed pales in comparison to how it feels to swim in it. Watching people die, and delivering bad news all day, every day takes an unmeasurable toll on a person. We chose a career in which we would be challenged and could help patients to live, not to watch people die one right after the other—for months on end. We are strong and built differently . . . or else we couldn't do the job in the first place. But everyone has a breaking point. We can only take so much pain and loss.

On top of this, the mental toll it takes to watch your coworkers struggle and then quit or leave to go travel and never come back is harder than it might seem on the outside. Critical care needs a team that is well-oiled, intimate, and trusting. If the team is constantly changing and disrupted, this adds another dynamic of exhaustion and hopelessness that is hard to describe. You need to be able to lean on your teammates at all levels of knowledge and specialties to do your job, even at the most basic level. Without this . . . there is an emotional and mental emptiness and loneliness that is hard to describe.

When all the faces and voices around you are unfamiliar, it's like you're taking on the world of death alone. It's essential that a team has an unshakable camaraderie during times like a pandemic. Unfortunately, this was undermined in many cases by the failure of hospitals to provide a basic level of security in terms of level of pay and safety.

The mask mandates were another contentious issue during the pandemic. While I understand the necessity of wearing a properly fitted N95 mask to prevent the transmission of COVID, the blanket mandate requiring the general public to wear *any* type of mask eventually became excessive.

Many of the homemade masks people wore provided little to no real protection. I recently had a discussion with one of our infectious disease doctors (who has been practicing medicine almost as long as I've been alive). He believed the mask mandates were largely unnecessary after the initial phase of the pandemic, once we had a clearer understanding of how the virus spread. Unless the government had been prepared to provide every American with an N95 mask and ensure proper fit testing, the mandates served more as a gesture than a scientifically sound measure.

Even Dr. Anthony Fauci, in early emails and statements, acknowledged that masks weren't particularly effective, especially the poor quality ones most people were wearing.[8] In that moment, at least, he was being honest.

That said, do masks work to some degree? Perhaps. I'm not so opposed to masks that I'd refuse to wear one where required, it comes with the territory of being a nurse. And I've never been condescending or judgmental toward those who choose to wear a mask; everyone has the right to make personal choices about their safety and comfort. (Unless you are in a car alone, then I'm judging you for sure.)

It's entirely possible that masks prevented cases of COVID, especially in settings where everyone wore them and maintained distance. However, there's also an argument to suggest that prolonged mask-wearing, especially in children, may have disrupted immune system development by limiting exposure to everyday pathogens.

In 2021, after a year of mandated mask-wearing, my kids' school district finally made masks optional. The reaction online was explosive. Facebook lit up with comments like, "You're putting my child's life at risk—this should be illegal," and, "This is unacceptable; we're in the middle of a pandemic, and decisions like this should be left to medical professionals."

Some parents even threatened to pull their children out of school.

Yet, ironically, schools had been the primary source of outbreaks in our community during the mandate. Why? Because kids, as much as they try, are not capable of consistently wearing masks properly. Even when they do, the level of protection is minimal at best. The psychological toll that masks took on children far outweighed the limited benefits they provided.

My own kids' behavior changed significantly while they were required to wear masks in school. They told me it was hard to participate in class, and they disliked not being able to see their friends' faces. My youngest even stopped talking in class altogether for a while, frustrated that no one could understand him through his mask.

If my kids felt silenced, I can only imagine that many others did too. Masks may have been a (mediocre) barrier against germs, but they also became a barrier to connection, expression, communication and learning.

Beyond my frustrations with the mask mandates, as I convey in Part I, what haunts me most about this pandemic is the way so many people died. Alone. It is unimaginable, and yet it became a tragic reality for countless families. Patients spent their final moments with no one but a nurse by their side. No family. No friends. Just the sterile walls of a hospital room and the sound of machines whirring and beeping.

The no-visitor policies that hospitals implemented were, in most cases, unforgiving. They didn't allow exceptions, even for those at the very end of their lives. Imagine being married for 50 years, and your spouse; your partner, your best friend—

contracts COVID. She becomes so sick that she's hospitalized, and it becomes clear she won't recover.

You are not allowed to be in the room to hold her hand, to kiss her forehead, or to say goodbye.

It's devastating. Devastation is the only word for it.

Shouldn't the decision to risk exposure be yours to make as a spouse or family member? Or does that responsibility lie with hospital administrators or government agencies? Personally, I know exactly where I stand. If my mother, father, or brother were dying in the ICU, security would have a hard time keeping me out of that room.

The loneliness, fear, and heartbreak that patients and their families endured due to these restrictions were unconscionable. Witnessing it shook me to my core, many times.

I understand that hospitals and governments were trying to manage a crisis, but in doing so, they stripped away one of the most fundamental aspects of humanity—being there for each other in our most vulnerable moment.

Barb's family in Part I having to make the decision over a screen of what to do with their dying loved one—this happened hundreds of times a day to COVID-suffering patients and their families. I know for a fact that if Barb's husband were allowed in the hospital, he would have been there holding her hand the entire time.

These laws were particularly infuriating because there were government officials sneaking out into public spaces, not wearing masks, and not abiding by their own rules. One great example was Governor Newsom in California, eating at the *French Laundry* restaurant in November 2020, with no mask on, in a large group of people, not following any of his restrictive COVID policies. Meanwhile, people across the nation were DYING ALONE because this disease was supposedly so deadly and horrible. If he could eat dinner with a large group of people, our patients should have been allowed *at least* one visitor if their death was imminent.

The privileged hypocrisy enrages me.

Similarly, it's ridiculous and offensive to me that so many people had to die alone in 2020/2021 yet now, in 2024, visitors are completely allowed in COVID patients' rooms! Hundreds of thousands of people died alone over FaceTime back then, but now visitors are allowed in to hold hands and hug and kiss and be there for their family members. What the hell was the point of all that nonsense? I don't understand it.

The overall lackadaisical attitude we now have in 2025 towards COVID is so completely opposite to the strict, terrified rules that we had in 2020/2021. This highlights how ridiculous the overreaction, the fear mongering, and the literal panic about this disease was. It still exists; it still kills people—why are there no visitor restrictions at all? What has changed about this disease and how it is spread that the attitude and policy can be so vastly different?

Listen, I get that these rules are put into place for a reason. I fully understand that the husband of the dying lady could contract the disease and end up spreading it to like 4,872 other people (or whatever). I hear that as a valid argument.

But here is the deal. If you are at a very high risk of dying from COVID because you are predisposed, have comorbidities, or are on an immune-suppressing medication, then STAY HOME. Stay away from the husband who just said goodbye to his dying wife. And if you can't stay home, then obtain proper protection like an N95 mask. Otherwise, rest easy knowing that this disease has rarely killed healthy people with no medical conditions to speak of. YES, I know that it has killed some otherwise healthy people. But *almost none* when compared to people with preexisting health issues.

There were doctors all over the globe who were trying to

get the attention of the media, the government, and the world, showing important data and trying to save lives. There were treatments that were being thrown out because they did not benefit specific people's pockets.

One of the only people in America who was not afraid to allow these people to speak on his public forum that I am aware of (and likely one reason his popularity soared during this period) was Joe Rogan. He seems to believe that experts—regardless of public political affiliation, or popular opinion—should be heard, considered, and allowed to speak. He gave several doctors and scientists on his show the chance to speak inconvenient truths about treatments, the behavior of the virus, and what we could do to stop it or lessen its impact. Unfortunately, none of these people were allowed on mainstream media because they went against the narrative created and protected by Tony Fauci, his media cronies, and the government.

That, folks, is a violation of our first amendment rights and should be condemned.

Right now, the two most common treatments for COVID are Paxlovid and Remdesivir. We currently still use Remdesivir in the ICU I work at. When I go to Google these drugs, the results I get when I search for Remdesivir are primarily from the drug manufacturer or national biomed companies. They all tout the amazing power of this drug, claiming that 89-95% of patients who take it recover and live.[9] There are a few types of websites that celebrate what a miracle drug this is.

However, if you look at the actual, published, verified scientific studies, they tell a very different story.

A few studies show that it can help to "clinically improve" patients, reduce recovery time and the number of "serious adverse events," but they also state that it has no effect on the mortality of patients.[10] In a 2020 editorial in the prestigious

Journal of the American Medical Association, McCreary and Angus literally state that there is no mortality difference between a placebo and Remdesivir.[11]

Huh.

It's therefore really interesting that, in March 2020, the manufacturer of Remdesivir (Gilead Sciences) struck a *one-billion-dollar* deal with the US and UK for it to become the leading treatment for COVID in our two nations.[12] Yet, when I search on the FDA's website (US Food and Drug Administration), there are no articles about how fantastic this treatment is, or how amazingly effective it is.

When I go to Google Ivermectin, though? Oh boyyy . . .

The very first site that pops up is the FDA. They are like, "Despite what you may have heard, this drug is dangerous and is NOT approved by us!!"[13]

But what does the actual science say?

One study states, "Randomized controlled treatment trials of Ivermectin in COVID-19 have found large, statistically significant reductions in mortality, time to clinical recovery, and time to viral clearance."[14]

Huh.

Ivermectin is cheap and readily available; why would we not use this as a primary treatment? It seems very suspicious to me that a drug with such high efficacy rates was debunked straight out of the gate, and a new, unproven drug is used instead. In most of the studies I have read about Ivermectin, they all state that there are "significant clinical research gaps" with this medication.[15]

Do you think it could be possible that the government put a blockade on this research for some reason? Because there are no such limitations on research on Remdesivir. My personal belief is that there is not enough funding given to researchers who want to study the effects of Ivermectin—or any other widely available drug with no patent to profit off—on a large scale, and this is why there are so few large-scale clinical trials started or completed.

I also encountered something on the ivermectin page of the FDA's website that left me both frustrated and baffled. There's a lovely article about how you should not take medication meant for animals (*this drug is also approved for humans, but thanks, government*). The article linked to "clinical trials" purportedly demonstrating the drug's ineffectiveness and potential dangers.[15] Intrigued, I clicked on several of these links, expecting clear, concise summaries of the findings. Instead, I found dense, convoluted reports that even as an educated and experienced medical professional, I struggled to decipher. I read through six different studies and came away unable to properly summarize or make sense of the data being presented.

The article continued, emphasizing in bold, underlined text that taking large doses of Ivermectin is NOT okay. While that may be a fair point, it raises an important question: why wasn't there better supported and adequately funded research conducted earlier? If proper studies had been prioritized, maybe people wouldn't have resorted to self-dosing or going to unreliable sources for guidance.

Instead, the drug appeared to be dismissed outright, leaving many to speculate about ulterior motives. On the other hand, it's hard to ignore the glaring support for other treatments, like Remdesivir, which seemed to have a convenient "in" with the government or influential individuals. *ahem* Fauci

When he had COVID, Joe Rogan was brave enough to take Ivermectin despite an onslaught of government and media criticism. Instead of acknowledging his recovery, headlines sensationalized the story with phrases like "Joe Rogan Takes Horse De-Wormer," which were designed to discredit both the man and the drug. Rogan openly refuted these claims on his widely popular podcast platform, stating, "I literally got this drug from a doctor, and it has been approved for, and won the Nobel Peace Prize for, its use by human beings. CNN has to know that what they are saying is a lie."

The result? Joe Rogan did not die. He took the medication prescribed to him, recovered quickly, and was back to full health before the controversy had a chance to quiet down. Ignoring his following of medical advice, taking a proven drug under supervision and quick recovery; the media chose to use the moment to shame Rogan and mock Ivermectin without regard for its potential merits.

What's most upsetting is the possibility that lives could have been saved if Ivermectin had been studied and utilized more thoroughly. In some countries, Ivermectin was a standard, affordable, and readily available treatment for COVID-19 patients. Reports from other countries indicated it had life-saving potential, particularly in the early stages of the disease.[16] Yet here, in one of the most advanced countries in the world, it was dismissed outright, and patients were denied access to a treatment that might have made a difference. What a total outrage. The entire situation is a frustrating example of how profit-motive, bureaucracy, misinformation, and misplaced priorities can interfere with effective healthcare.

Vaccines are a whole other topic of conversation that I could write an entire book on. As of 2024, in my personal experience, I saw almost no difference in hospitalizations and deaths between vaccinated and non-vaccinated patients in real life. I had to ask if people were vaccinated upon admission to the ICU, and while more people overall were vaccinated, there were plenty of them in the hospital with COVID.

When the vaccines first came out, people unwilling to get one were being shamed, cancelled, and bullied. The government was effectively saying that if you didn't get a vaccine, you were part of the problem and were essentially killing other people.

The problem here is that there was almost no data to refer to. There were very few—if any— fully published and peer-reviewed studies on these shots. They were granted "emergent use" by the WHO (World Health Organization) and the FDA because people were panicking (or made to panic) about COVID.

The amount of fear put into the hearts of Americans was astronomical.

So, when the vaccines came out, despite the lack of evidence, the pressure to get one was extreme. There was so little data on the long-term ramifications of the vaccines that many people were understandably wary of it. Robert F Kennedy Jr. reports in his book *The Real Anthony Fauci*, that he believes that vaccine injuries by that point had been under-reported by approximately 80%![16] This suggests that these vaccines are not as safe as we are being told they are.

One of my friends was pregnant during all of this. She worked for our hospital system, which was mandating these vaccines for all healthcare professionals. She did not feel safe or comfortable injecting her body while pregnant with a medication that was not thoroughly researched. At this point, there were no studies that showed the effects of these shots on pregnant women, their unborn child, or the pregnancy overall.

She attempted to get a medical excuse, but no OB-GYN in our area would give her one. They all kept saying, "We are being told to tell you that it is likely safe, and that many pregnant women who have gotten the vaccine have gone on to give birth to healthy children without issues."

She pleaded her case to at least three different doctors. Not one would give her the medical excuse.

She refused to get the vaccine and was fired, despite having worked there for nearly 20 years.

The only reason I got vaccinated was to keep my job. I needed employment like most people, and as a nurse, it was almost impossible to get or keep a job in healthcare if you weren't vaccinated. I waited until the very last day before I would be fired, hoping and praying that they would drop the mandate.

My main concern was the lack of data on women of childbearing age and what it would do to my ability to have children. At the time, I largely felt my days of having children were behind me, but a small part of me still wondered. And I didn't want this vaccine to be the reason I could never have kids again. In the end, I decided to get it because I felt like I had no choice.

It was a terrible feeling. I felt like I was being forced to do something against my will, I felt disempowered from making decisions about my body.

Once the vaccines rolled out, despite their promise to protect us, not many of the rules changed. We were still terrified of it; people were still dying and it didn't seem that vaccination made a huge difference in the number of deaths.

As of this writing, approximately 70% of the American population is "fully vaccinated."[17]

What does this mean, exactly?

Well, it just means that you've completed the recommended number of doses, which varies with each brand of shot. It is estimated that a 90% or higher vaccination rate is needed for the true "herd immunity" that everyone was so concerned about in 2021/2022.[18] So, the argument that COVID-19 death rates fell because herd immunity was achieved through vaccination is patently false.

As of May 2023, CMS (Center for Medicare & Medicaid Services—the government agency that places rules and regulations on healthcare facilities getting reimbursed by government funds) redacted their vaccine mandate.[19] They no longer require that all healthcare workers in funded facilities be vaccinated. This is very interesting, as it indicates to me that the vaccines do not work like they said they do, they are not necessary for herd immunity, and that COVID is not really a concern at all anymore.

The CDC stopped keeping track of the COVID-19 deaths as of September 2023. Their website states that from March 2020 until September 2023, 1,143,724 people died from COVID in the United States.[20] If you do the math, with our current population of around 333 million people, 1.14 million is about 0.34%.

Now, with the benefit of hindsight in 2025, we can look at this data and see that COVID absolutely did not do the damage that the government kept saying it would.

To give this more context, heart disease alone killed 0.2% of our population in 2023.[21] If you go to the CDC website and add all the deaths from heart disease from 2020–2023, you get a number around 2.8 million.[22] That is 0.83% of our national population; almost one-and-a-half times the amount of people that COVID killed.

Where is the national outrage? Our current diet of processed, poisonous food is rarely talked about by the CDC or the media. Why? We are dying from heart disease at a rate of almost double that of COVID. We deserve answers as to why there was such utter panic and destruction of our nation over this disease, but not over a disease that is objectively worse and more burdensome on our country.

It's important to remember that these numbers of COVID deaths do not take into account the amount of people who died *incidentally* with a positive COVID test. I saw this many times with my own eyes.

Someone would come into the hospital with a severe and late complication from diabetes and unfortunately pass away, but their medical record would show that COVID was the cause of death. I have heard of several doctors who literally left their profession because they could not tolerate this fraud. These patients were dying—and yes, they tested positive for COVID—but they did not die *from* it.

So, the real death toll is likely much lower than what has been reported by the CDC.

Nowadays COVID is usually treated as a bad cold. The panic has evaporated. People who have lots of medical problems can still be greatly affected by COVID but, honestly, not much more than they could be by traditional pneumonia. In the hospital, we still put COVID-positive patients on airborne precautions, but we don't do this with pneumonia patients.

We are still acting like this disease is as bad as tuberculosis, one of the deadliest contagious diseases in history. Even if this were true, do you know what else spreads by airborne means? Pneumonia. The common cold. Respiratory syncytial virus (RSV). Measles. We do not have as severe precautions for these as we do for COVID.

Why?

The lack of outrage over the misrepresentation of this pandemic's severity is also deeply concerning to me. Far too often, we accept numbers and narratives at face value, rarely pausing to question their origins or accuracy. Most of us choose instead to place blind trust in figures of authority like Dr. Fauci and the institutions behind him.

The reality is that much of the data we were fed—death counts, infection rates, and projections—was inflated, manipulated, or misreported. Why? Was it fear of government retribution? Pressure from unseen powers? Or simply the inner workings of a system built to perpetuate its own authority? The motivations remain unclear. What I do know is this: we, as a nation, were not told the full truth.

What troubles me most is that, while many other countries focused on treating their patients, using effective, accessible therapies, and moving forward; we became paralyzed. We politicized the virus, turned science into a weapon of division, and left the American people drowning in fear and misinformation. While much of the rest of the world adapted, treated, and began to recover; we lingered in a state of confusion and distrust.

To the families who lost loved ones to COVID-19, please know this: I see your pain, and I grieve with you. I wish with every fiber of my being that things could have been different. I wish we could have saved them all. I wish the circumstances surrounding their care had been free from the politics, profit motives, and misinformation that clouded so much of the pandemic response.

I also want to express my deepest respect for the healthcare professionals who fought tirelessly on the front lines. Those who bravely spoke out about effective treatments, preventative measures, and the evolving science—only to be dismissed, silenced, or ignored. Their courage deserved to be celebrated, their voices heard, their advice followed. Instead, they were drowned by a relentless narrative that prioritized fear over truth and profits over patients.

This was a pandemic of loss. Not just of lives, which was devastating in itself, but the loss of trust in our healthcare system, in our leaders, and in the institutions we are meant to rely on in times of crisis. The choices made by those in power, the media, corporations, and government agencies, undoubtedly cost lives.

If only we had been guided by transparency and integrity

rather than by fear and greed, how many more people could we have saved?

To those mourning a loved one, I offer my sincerest condolences. Your loss is immeasurable, and I am so sorry for the pain you've endured. I am also sorry for the loss healthcare itself has suffered—a loss of trust, unity, and direction that will likely take years, if not decades, to heal.

What a shame.

What a tragedy.

But I hold on to hope that we can learn from these mistakes and demand better—not just for ourselves, but for the future of healthcare and for every life that depends on it.

CHAPTER 2

BURNOUT

THE BREAKING POINT OF CARE

HEALTHCARE WORKERS' lives have been affected by the pandemic in a tragic way. We are the front lines of this shitshow.

It makes me think a lot about the Army infantry, the "front-line fighters" in a war. They get all amped-up to kill the bad guy, and they are the first to get gunned down, killed, maimed, or otherwise greatly affected by the actions of war. That's us. Except we don't have the backup that the Army does. They have the Marines, Navy, and Air Force that will come swooping in to back them up and save the day.

Saying we are on the "front line" implies that there are people on the "back line." It implies that we have support that will step in when we cannot go on. But we do not have that.

A study by Rotenstein et al. noted that, as of 2023, 50% of all healthcare workers are dangerously burnt out.[1]

Many of us are suffering with the "war wounds" of depression, anxiety, compassion fatigue, disrupted home lives, mental exhaustion, brain fog, burnout, chronic stress, physical fatigue, and a chronic sense of unfulfillment. Especially as we are in the wake of a pandemic and still feeling its effects daily. But burnout is rampant even without a pandemic.

Healthcare burnout is not just bad for healthcare workers; it is associated with an exponential increase in clinical errors.[2] Nurses are expected to be where the buck stops to prevent medication errors, but when we are this burnt-out, the chances of making a mistake are much higher.

Yes, I know it's not the same as being shot at or bombed. But we did not sign up to be shot at. We signed up to spend years of schooling to have long, fulfilling, challenging, well-paid careers. I mean, we all knew coming out of nursing school or medical school that life on the wards can get hairy and stressful occasionally, even daily. But not *every* minute of *every* shift forever and ever. That wasn't part of the deal.

And it just keeps getting worse.

Nurses are experiencing burnout on an unprecedented scale. Historically, when burnout set in, nurses had the option to shift specialties for a fresh start. Worked in the ICU for two years? Maybe it's time to try cardiac nursing for a new challenge. Spent 13 years on a medical-surgical (med-surg) team? A switch to rehab might be refreshing!

But now, there's no escaping the chaos, and switching specialties no longer provides a break. ICU nurses find cardiac nursing equally overwhelming, and med-surg nurses stepping into rehab discover it's just as—if not more—ridiculous.

We're trapped in a system that never lightens the load, no matter where we go or how hard we try to adapt. And so, we're leaving. Nurses are walking away from bedside care in droves. What was once celebrated as "The Year of the Nurse" in 2020 has, by 2024, become "The Year of 'Eff This, I'm Out'" for healthcare professionals.

I work with a woman who has been a nurse for over twenty-five years. She has been at the same hospital for almost all her career, and she is just as burnt out as the rest of us. But she will tell you that it was never like this back in the day. Even as recently as fifteen to twenty years ago—the mid 2000s—nursing was simpler, less intrusive in your home life, and demanded less responsibility overall.

She also told me that there used to be a lot more backup, mainly as there were lots more CNAs (certified nursing assistants). This made the workload much more tolerable. She commented that nurses have had to take on more and more of the increased burden and responsibility in healthcare. And yet, she says, we are respected less and less, by patients, their families, and even doctors.

Her main complaint now is how patients and their families treat her. She is a take-no-shit type of woman (a classic nursing archetype) and yet is still spoken to like she's an idiot, yelled at, and physically abused. It is unbearable. This treatment, combined with the added responsibility, has her on the verge of retiring early, which would decrease her benefits in retirement. What a shame it would be to lose this excellent and experienced nurse because of burnout.

I recently saw a tweet that said, "Why I prefer the term *exploitation* over *burnout*: burnout makes it about workers' feelings. Exploitation draws our attention to employer practices and policies which require structural solutions."[3]

This is an important delineation; burnout is real, and employees' feelings—especially in healthcare—get all messed up and raw after a while.

But exploitation? Exploitation is also *super real*. Hospitals, with rare exceptions, literally do not care about you personally; and you need to make sure that you are taking care of yourself first. Being aware of this is so important. Being exploited for years on end as a healthcare worker takes its toll, and it is a clear sign of a systemic failure in which human beings are the main victims.

I think burnout, at least to some degree, is common in almost all jobs and professions. You can only do something for so long over and over until you get a little sick of it.

My generation is much more conscious of this, and we have less tolerance for misery. Our grandparents stayed in the same shitty job for 145 years and retired making $4 more an hour than when they started and were thankful for it. But if you look at the numbers, they were (by and large) earning a decent wage and able to afford to live off one income doing that. They could go work for the mill on a production line, and stay there for a 35-year career, and still be able to feed their families and afford to buy a house and car.

Now? LOL! If there aren't two incomes in a family and you didn't buy a house before 2021, you get to enjoy a lifetime of watching your rent go up by ten percent each year while—if you're lucky—your income goes up one to two per cent. For most professions, it is virtually impossible to survive off one full-time income. This compounds the burnout in many ways, not least because you feel you aren't even being compensated fairly for all of your efforts!

Merriam-Webster's Dictionary defines burnout as "exhaustion of physical or emotional strength or motivation, usually resulting from prolonged stress or frustration."[4]

I would like you to pay close attention to the "as a result of prolonged stress or frustration" part of this definition. Being in healthcare is stressful most of the time. Being a floor nurse on a med-surg unit, ER, ICU, or almost any other specialty is like going into battle every day, except that battle is full of piss, shit, blood, screaming, arguing, and mental exhaustion, all while trying to think critically and not kill anyone.

The "frustration" part of this definition is key to me.

Patients are horrible 80% of the time. Take Jerry in the first part of this book. He is unhealthy and takes no responsibility or accountability for the situation he finds himself in, and instead instinctively and mindlessly takes out all his emotions, frustrations and fears on the healthcare staff.

Many patients are so awful, I cannot even express it to you, but I have dedicated an entire chapter of this book to the subject. It is *incredibly* frustrating to work with patients like this. It is incredibly frustrating to continually feel that you don't have the backup and support you need to do your job well. Even if you work in a good hospital system where you do feel supported, the frustration level can still be extreme when dealing with patients and their families.

Imagine going to work every day, having people's actual lives in your hands, and being disrespected, spoken down to, questioned in every imaginable way, physically assaulted, and verbally abused. Imagine doing all of that while simultaneously being so careful and scared to not make a single error because someone could literally die from it.

"Exhaustion" does not even begin to cut it.

I want to be very clear that I understand not all areas of nursing/healthcare are awful. I am also very aware that not all places in which nurses/healthcare workers work suck. There are some nurses who love their careers and their workplace and don't have much to complain about. But I also know that, even though I work in a place in which I mostly feel I have backup and support, and I mostly feel heard and listened to, I am STILL burnt out. I am still exhausted. Some days are better than others, but I am still completely over dealing with some patients and their family members.

This is the nature of the job in 95% of cases.

Talking about burnout leads us to the ongoing joke that is "self-care for healthcare professionals." All the self-care guides on the internet are geared towards people who have nine-to-five, Monday–Friday jobs, or jobs from home that they do on their computers. Never, in the six million hours that I've spent reading or listening to self-help books (don't judge me), have I come across ONE self-help program specifically for shift-working healthcare workers.

We need help. We need resources. One of my future goals is to write a book or program designed to help shift workers take better care of themselves.

It's hard to understand the toll of shift work unless you've done it. And let me tell you, as a healthcare professional, it gets old pretty quick. You're expected to be constantly thinking critically, looking out for errors, following up on tasks, and staying alert for twelve hours straight.

Sounds doable, right? Maybe if you're a robot. But for actual humans? It's madness. I don't know a single nurse in the hospital who gets an uninterrupted lunch break. Not one. The reality is, you're lucky if you can wolf down half a stale sandwich while standing at the nurses' station, charting patient updates with one hand.

This is not natural. Humans weren't designed to be awake, focused, and responsible for people's lives for twelve hours straight, day after day, night after night. It's no wonder by the end of three shifts in a row (or God forbid, more), you're basically a zombie masquerading as a human.

I've done seven shifts in a row before. Seven. By the end of that marathon, I was so mentally fried and physically depleted I couldn't even think straight. The first day off after a stretch like that isn't really a day off—it's a recovery mission. You're so drained you can barely function. Sure, you might manage to run an errand or stumble into the gym, but most of the day is spent horizontal, either rotting on the couch or in bed, staring blankly at a screen and contemplating your life choices.

The second and third days off? Better, but not great. Just when you start feeling human again, the fourth day hits, and you're already psyching yourself up for the next round of shifts.

Now, imagine trying to manage all this while also raising kids. Because, you know, days off as a parent are never actually "days off." My mornings still start early, getting the kids to school, followed by after-school activities, errands, and housework. Somewhere in the chaos, I'm supposed to squeeze in "self-care"—ha! Good luck with that.

The truth is, I can probably count on one hand the number of days in a year I get to sleep in or truly relax. And while I fully accept that my choice to have kids plays a huge role in this insanity, I also know I'm not alone in feeling this way. Every shift worker I talk to agrees: it's exhausting.

Sure, there are perks to shift work. I can attend a random school performance in the middle of the day or make it to a parent-teacher conference without having to take time off. And, yes, going to Target at 10 am on a Tuesday instead of battling the Saturday crowd is nice. But let's be real: at least for me, those small conveniences don't come close to making up for the logistical nightmares shift work creates.

On workdays, I leave the house at 6:15 am and don't get home until nearly 8 pm. Finding childcare that accommodates those hours is practically impossible. Most daycares don't open until 7 am—and forget about them transporting your kids to school. After-school care? Sure, but most close at 7 pm, leaving me scrambling for the last 45 minutes. If you have a partner to help, great. If you don't—or if they're also a shift worker—you're basically stuck trying to clone yourself.

What makes this all even harder is the complete lack of institutional support for healthcare workers. I was talking to a night-shift nurse recently and asked her what she thought the biggest challenge of nursing was. Without hesitation, she said,

"The lack of support and the outright dismissal of our need for self-care. They act like they care, but the second you try to take time off, you're shamed for it."

She's absolutely right. Paid time off is essential in a job as grueling as healthcare, but instead of being encouraged to use it, we're made to feel guilty for needing it. It's like, "Sure, take care of yourself, but if you do, expect some guilting and maybe even a lecture when you get back."

And then there's the truly absurd part: when the resources that are supposed to help us are taken away. My hospital used to have an Employee Assistance Program (EAP) that offered counseling, emotional support, and other resources to help us manage the stress of the job. Sounds great, right? Well, in 2021, they canceled it.

Let me say that again: in the middle of a global health crisis, they decided to eliminate the one program designed to support the mental health of their employees. If that's not a slap in the face, I don't know what is.

The result? Healthcare workers are burning out and leaving the profession in droves. It's not that we don't care about our patients—we care deeply. But the constant demands, lack of support, and sheer exhaustion are driving us to a breaking point. Many of us don't want to leave, but we feel like we have no other choice. And here's the kicker: this isn't just a problem for us. It's a problem for everyone.

When nurses, doctors, techs, and CNAs leave healthcare, the entire system suffers. There aren't enough of us to care for patients, and the weight on those who remain becomes unbearable. It's a vicious cycle.

And here's the stark truth: this crisis will affect *every single American*. When there aren't enough healthcare workers left to care for the sick, injured, and vulnerable, it won't just be our problem—it'll be everyone's problem. The care people take for granted won't be there when they need it most. We need change, and we need it now.

If we don't start supporting healthcare workers in meaningful ways—through better policies, better resources, and a hell of a lot more respect—this system will collapse. And when it does, the ripple effects will touch every community, every family, and every individual in this country.

Healthcare burnout isn't just a personal issue. It's a societal one. And if we continue to ignore it, the consequences will be devastating.

CHAPTER 3

BEHIND THE SCRUBS
THE UNSEEN TOLL OF ABUSE IN HEALTHCARE

I MENTIONED I was writing a book to some fellow nurses. They asked what it was about, and I told them it was about how the healthcare system in America is going to shit.

Every person within earshot nodded their heads.

I spoke about how healthcare is now much more about customer service than about making people well and fixing their medical problems. I said that COVID had really fucked up our world and that being a nurse would never be the same.

But when I got to one topic, everyone really perked up.

I started to talk about the behavior of patients and their families. I said that ever since the so-called 'patient satisfaction-dictatorship' program began—a term I use to refer to the initiative launched by the Centers for Medicare and Medicaid Services (CMS) in the early 2000s to tie hospital reimbursements to patient satisfaction scores—patients have started behaving like complete animals most of the time."

"This building is NOT a hotel," I said, "it's a HOSPITAL."

The nurse sitting next to me, said, "YES. There's an 'H' on the side of this building, and patients think it stands for 'hotel'!"

Oh, how right she is.

In 2002, CMS began developing a "patient satisfaction program" (officially, the Hospital Consumer Assessment of Healthcare Providers and Systems, or HCAHPS), requiring hospitals to send surveys to patients after medical encounters. All hospitals reimbursed by CMS under the Inpatient Prospective Payment System had to comply, with the aim of gathering patient feedback to drive focused improvements in medical care. CMS was touting this as a major quality improvement tool that would benefit hospitals, with no downsides.

In 2006, CMS launched the nationwide HCAHPS survey, making patient-reported experience a key part of hospital evaluation and public reporting. Bland et al. reviewed the purpose of these surveys and their effectiveness at encouraging improvement. They stated in their 2022 review, "The original survey development stemmed from the movement toward health care consumerization. This involved framing the person using health care services as a consumer to be satisfied, rather than a patient at the receiving end of whatever doctors thought best."[1]

The growth of this mindset of healthcare consumerism (or "pleasing the patient") has been both beneficial and detrimental to American healthcare.

In an idealistic world, these surveys show healthcare providers where they need to improve and offer a relatively cheap way of accessing this information. We can send a survey out, and within a matter of weeks or days, can then add data to a database and see where we are trending in each area of healthcare. If someone has an emergency surgery, for example, and feels like he was not listened to by his providers and was in extreme, unrelieved pain for hours on end, the facility would get feedback from him on his survey and be able to improve from there. Theoretically.

However, the reality is very different.

What we see in the real world is that patients use this mindset of consumerism and "pleasing the patient" in a negative way. Instead of getting genuine feedback, these survey results are fraught with drama, emotions, and vendettas. Let's say someone is told information about their health they don't like. It is not uncommon for this to provoke them to only provide negative feedback—*even if* they had a great hospital stay with no major issues.

Because of distortions and biases like these, the results of these surveys are not reliable enough to initiate change within our broken healthcare system. It seems to me that more resources are spent on educating facility staff on how to get good survey results than on how to provide better care. I have sat through many staff training sessions, for example, where they give us specific stock phrases to use when responding to patient questions that are directly aimed at increasing patient satisfaction scores. Many patients are aware of the power they hold through these surveys and use them as a weapon to express dissatisfaction—such as over wait times, billing disputes, or personal grievances—not as a tool to initiate improvements within the system.

It has become a penalty system for healthcare workers, not a path to healthcare improvement.

This mindset shift has come with an increase in terrible behavior by patients towards the people who care for them. This has been a huge change over the last 20 years, and I feel has gotten exponentially worse in the last five years.

I work with a nurse who has been in the field for almost 30 years. She says that patients in the 1990s and early 2000s *almost never* acted the way they do now. She has told me stories of how, if a patient was acting aggressive or horrible, they assumed there was a clinical reason for it because *people didn't just act like assholes for no reason*. She believes that the level of entitlement of patients has quadrupled since she started as a nurse, and that it has gotten worse the more we have focused on patient satisfaction. It was very rare in her early days, she says, that nurses were physically, mentally or verbally abused by patients. However, when such incidents did occur—as is still often the case today—nurses were told to "get over it," and action was rarely taken.

In my 15 years, I have had more miserable, grouchy, angry, verbally abusive, physically abusive, and downright *mean* patients than I have had nice, thankful, and sweet patients. Not just a little bit rude— giving me attitude because I didn't get to their room within 0.00001 seconds of their pressing their call button—I'm talking straight-up awful.

An example? Sure. How about the guy who would grab tightly onto my hand or arm as soon as I went near him—regardless of what I was going to do or the amount of forewarning I gave him? Not just grab tightly because he was scared but *squeeze* specifically to hurt me while muttering hateful shit under his breath.

Or how about the patient who, any time I went near her, would try to kick me while telling me to "get the fuck away" from her?

Or maybe the male patient who told me there was no way I could possibly be competent since I was a girl and "couldn't be older than 17" (I was 38 at the time).

Oh, there was also the guy who told me that I was a "fucking cunt" because I wouldn't give him Dilaudid (hydromorphone, a potent opioid) every time he wanted it. Which was a lot of the time.

Then there was the man who would throw anything he could get his hands on at any member of staff that walked into his room.

I've had patients deliberately spit at me, try to bite me, actually bite me, twist my arm so hard my skin broke, try to head-butt me, kick at me, try to swing at my face, and try to rip off my shirt. We even had a patient *pick up her bedside table* and throw it at a nurse.

I have had patients belittle me, tell me I am stupid, call me names like cunt, bitch, fucking asshole, twat, dumbass . . . the list could go on for pages. I have had patients look at me in the eye and ask for a man because women don't know what they're talking about. I have had patients legitimately *scream* at me over something as simple as water. More than one nurse I've talked to has told me that they have had a patient incessantly push their call bell because they want ice, when they are in the next room coding a person and literally watching them die.

In Part I, Jerry continuously presses his call bell to ask for his pain meds. He is not an addict. He does not have mental health issues. He is an oriented grown man. And yet he still harasses the nurses nonstop for something he knows is unavailable to him. Mildred's daughter is rude, disrespectful, and pushy to a person that she does not even know because that person is caring for her mom. And this person is just supposed to "take it" and get over it.

According to the American Hospital Association (AHA), in 2022, 44% of nurses reported being physically assaulted on the job, and 68% reported being verbally abused.[2] That means four out of ten nurses taking care of someone are being *physically harmed* just by doing their jobs, and seven out of ten are being *emotionally and mentally tormented*.

This is unacceptable.

When a patient or family member is being erratic and violent, either physically or verbally, healthcare workers cannot do their jobs. We cannot take care of your mother if you are absolutely losing your mind in the room or hallway. If we are scared for our own personal mental or physical well-being, we cannot do our jobs.

One time, I had a patient's nephew asking for water for his uncle. We had told him multiple times that the patient was NPO (couldn't have anything by mouth). He continued to stand in the hallway and *yell* that we are all lazy bitches and don't do shit, and to get off our asses and help his uncle. We had to call security because he was so belligerent, and then he started to physically threaten us, saying he doesn't give a shit about security because he has been in jail before, saying he would "fuck you all up if I want to."

This is verbal abuse and a physical threat. It is totally uncalled for, and charges should have been pressed. But because he walked away with security, we were just supposed to get back to work.

There are few laws protecting healthcare workers from abuse. The main problem with laws surrounding abuse is that patients and their families usually end up claiming that they were not in their right mind because of illness and/or trauma they endured. Court cases are often thrown out based on an assumption that healthcare workers basically "signed up" for dealing with people at their worst. The treatment of healthcare workers is swept under the rug and ignored because it just comes with the territory.

I have personally been attacked and verbally abused countless times but have never been able to follow through to do anything about it.

My sister-in-law is an RN, and she had a patient who told her he was going to come back to the hospital and shoot her with an AR15 semi-automatic rifle. He faced no consequences. In my opinion, he should be jailed for a threat that severe. Instead, he's chilling at home now because his *life was saved*.

The AHA and some related healthcare institutions are

trying to pass a bill called the Safety from Violence for Healthcare Employees (SAVE) Act, which would give healthcare workers the same protections that flight attendants, flight crews, and airport staff have.[3] This would make it a federal crime, for example, if you put your hands on a healthcare worker.

No, this legislation would not change everything, but it would start the process of shifting blame from the victims to the perpetrators, where it belongs. I do not give any shits that you are having the worst day of your life—you have NO RIGHT to assault or abuse me or any of my coworkers in any way. There's a difference between being cold and discourteous because you're having a bad time versus getting violent or threatening me if you don't get what you want.

Let's be very clear here, your grandma didn't get her pain medications when she demanded them, not because she didn't scream loudly enough at me, but because they weren't due for another two hours. We have protocols in place to make sure patients don't *die from an overdose*, not because we enjoy torturing them or like getting yelled at. And trust me, if you throw something at me, or kick at me, you are NOT more likely to get what you want in a timely manner. It actually puts you in danger because I am *far less* likely to go into your room after you do something like that to me, and I could possibly miss something which could result in a complication to your health.

(Also, a side note, if you are able to scream at me in anger, your pain level likely isn't as high as you say it is.)

The abuse is so frequent that when a patient is *actually nice* to one of us, we literally run to the nurses' station to talk about it. "OMG! Can you believe how NICE the man in room six is?? He even said THANK YOU when I gave him his medicine today!"

"Oh, the patient in room three is so sweet . . . she said she appreciates everything we're doing for her and said that the world is lucky to have a nurse like me."

Like, seriously . . . healthcare workers get *excited* because a patient says thank you for providing them medical care and potentially/likely saving their lives?

Dang.

The level of expectation and sense of entitlement of patients and their family is completely out of control and beyond any sense of dignity. Ever since word got out that hospitals and healthcare facilities are required to ensure your "stay is pleasurable" and that you "got everything you needed and requested" while hospitalized, patients' behavior has become more and more outrageous.

Are we trying to make these people healthy or make them happy? Because I know a lovely massage parlor down the street that will do the second, if that's what they're after.

This culture built around patient satisfaction must change, or there will be no more nurses, doctors, respiratory therapists, phlebotomists, CNAs—or any other support staff—to take care of these patients. The surveys themselves aren't the problem; they are a legitimate tool to gather useful data. The problem is the culture shift that has surrounded them in the medical community. We prioritize survey outcomes over medical outcomes; consumerism over health.

Granted, patients are caught in a broken system, but what I don't think they realize is, *so are we*. Somehow, their illnesses have become not just our responsibility, but our *fault*.

"Oh yeah, last time I was in here they didn't fix me right, so here I am again!"

Um, no sir, it is because you didn't take your diuretic pills because you don't want to pee all the time, so now you are drowning in your own fluids.

How has it become our responsibility to magically fix all of these people who do not listen to medical advice?

Here is an actual conversation I had with a patient:

> ME: Ma'am, you were instructed before leaving the hospital to take insulin three times a day to control your sugar levels to help your wound heal. You were also told that you need to increase your protein intake by drinking sugar-free protein shakes every day.
>
> PATIENT: Yeah, they told me that last time and I did it, but my wounds are getting worse!
>
> Oh no! Well, what was your sugar this morning?
>
> I didn't take it. I'm sick of sticking my fingers.
>
> Oh . . . okay . . . well, when did you last take your sugar level?
>
> I don't know, maybe three days ago?
>
> Uh . . . well what was it then?
>
> How am I supposed to remember that far back? I think it was like 250 or something.
>
> Alrighty then. But you've been taking your insulin three times a day as ordered?
>
> Um, NO, I just told you I'm sick of being poked. Now how come my wound is not healing?
>
> Your wound is not healing because you're not controlling your diabetes. Have you at least been drinking the protein supplements?
>
> No, those things are gross, but I did treat myself to some Wendy's the other day with my tax refund!

> ME: . . . .

Of course, not all patients are horrible. I have had some wonderful, kind and appreciative patients throughout my years as a nurse. I currently have a couple thank-you notes on my fridge from patients who wanted to express their gratitude. I have been given small gifts as little tokens of thanks. I had one patient who cried from appreciation every time I walked into her room. I've been invited to holiday celebrations, birthday parties, and funerals.

When I was doing home visits, I had an old man in his 80s who would dress up in a literal suit for my visits. When I asked him why he was always so dressed up, he said, "My dad taught me to have the utmost respect for someone who cares for me, and one way I can show that is by being properly prepared and put together for your arrival."

I mean, really?

And yet I have Mr. Meth in room ten telling me I am a piece-of-shit bitch who should go to hell for asking him to take his pills.

We see patients when they are in pain, confused, scared, angry, and hurt. Sometimes they are all of these at once. I also understand that many diseases, such as encephalopathies, can cause severe behavioral disturbances.[*] (I mention encephalopathy as it can turn the sweetest person into a demon.)

I am fully aware that suffering with these physical conditions and feelings make it very difficult (if not impossible) to be chipper and want to talk about sunshine and rainbows. When

---

[*] Encephalopathy: Any disorder, disease, such as infection, or damage affecting the brain's structure or function.

you are in ceaseless pain, or feel like you might die, it is hard to be nice to people.

But at the very least, *apologize* for when you were being terrible! I had a patient who spent most of my 36-hour shift being awful and hateful towards me and all the other staff. But towards the end of the shift, he grabbed my hand gently said, "I'm sorry I was so terrible to you . . . I just don't deal with pain well."

I recently had an emergency appendectomy and was in the worst pain of my entire life. I have given birth to two kids at home with no meds, so I have a pretty high pain tolerance. Both my husband and I thought I was dying because I was in so much pain and was so sick. Not once was I rude to staff. My pain was uncontrolled in the ER for about two hours. But I still never yelled at the people taking care of me.

When patients come to the hospital, or need some kind of healthcare, they are generally pretty sick. It means that there is a major dysfunction in their body requiring intervention to fix. That means they probably feel terrible, are in pain, and aren't acting like themselves. All of this is understandable. All healthcare professionals are trained in how to decipher patient behavior. We are taught to see through their anger and notice that it is (usually) fear.

We experience people break down sobbing in our arms when they suddenly have a realization that they are terrified and feel out of control. Like Jerry—eventually we see that he is just terrified and ashamed of himself. And despite the barrage of verbal abuse he had subjected me to, I sat next to him, listened to his concerns, and had an honest conversation. We understand, but there must be limits on how horribly people are allowed to treat healthcare workers.

Hospitals and other healthcare facilities and agencies outright discourage their employees from seeking legal recourse against a patient who physically assaults them. Their common excuses include: "They aren't in their right mind," "It must be their medications," "They are just in pain and scared," and "It's part of what you signed up for when you became a nurse."

Listen here, Cynthia, I absolutely did NOT sign up for getting kicked in the abdomen by an 80-pound aggressive alcoholic drug addict who doesn't want me suctioning her endotracheal tube. Nor did I sign up for Mr. Meth telling me what a "cunty bitch" I am. Nor for trying to keep Mr. Vodkalover in his bed while he calls me names and tries to literally rip my hand off of my arm.

That is actually not at all what I signed up for.

Healthcare professionals should be immediately backed up by administration and management if abuse of any type occurs.

I have stood *many* times in a manager's office, in or close to tears, relaying abuse I have endured. Many of these instances turn into the abuser complaining about me or my care, purely because they are not getting exactly what they want from me. Every time, I was told to brush it off because it's not a "big deal." The best outcome I have had is that I am taken off the patient's case, but that usually just leads to another nurse being abused.

How far would it actually have to go, I wonder, for it to be a big deal?

If a person assaults an airline or airport employee, it is over for them. Regardless of whether they're on drugs, or they have serious mental health issues, or they're sick. They would certainly be arrested and charged.

What is the difference between an airline uniform and scrubs that make them more of a priority to keep safe? How can we change this narrative that the ER is a place to be out-of-control, but the airport is a place to be respectable?

One way is to allow hospital and healthcare employees to

press charges and hold their patients accountable for better behavior. If a patient puts their hands on you, you should feel completely comfortable pressing all the charges possible, and you should be supported by management throughout. If we change our internal expectations of employees, eventually patients will begin to change.

We have a "red flag warning" in our system at my hospital that will pop up a warning that says, "Patient has a history of physical violence toward staff." That way we know to be on our toes while in that patient's room. This seems crazy to me; that physical assault towards healthcare workers is rampant enough in our society that we have a premade button in our medical record system for it.

Hospitals and healthcare facilities need to start holding their patients and their families accountable for their behavior towards staff, and laws need to change so that if someone is assaultive to healthcare workers, they can be legally blacklisted from certain medical establishments. I understand that even violent people may need life-saving treatment. However, if it became standard practice to hold people accountable for abusive behavior—making it clear that such actions could jeopardize their own care—they might begin to reconsider how they treat us.

Patients lie, cajole, manipulate, blame, and persecute innocent healthcare workers for their own ignorance and unwillingness to care for themselves. Not only do we carry the exhausting burden of caring for people during the most traumatic moments of their lives, but we are also unfairly blamed and shamed for the consequences of another adult's inability or failure to take care of themselves.

Patients should be held to higher standards, and there should be absolutely zero tolerance for violence or abuse of any kind against healthcare workers.

CHAPTER 4

NURSES' PROVERBIAL PLATES

THIS CHAPTER DISCUSSES the responsibilities of being a modern nurse and thereby the main reason why many nurses want to leave the profession.

Here are the responsibilities of a nurse for a typical shift on a medical-surgical floor—this is your standard, normal workload for the five to seven patients that you have assigned to you. I am not exaggerating. I wish that I were. They include:

1. Ensure that medications are ordered correctly by verifying they make sense along with the dose, timing, and disease process.
2. Call the doctor to correct medication orders if an error is found. (*This happens so frequently it's terrifying! I have caught hundreds of medication errors by doctors—we are the ones preventing a potentially deadly interaction, overdose, or low dose.*)
3. Find another nurse to double-check high-risk medications (like insulin or blood products).

4. Administer medications up to every single hour (or more if the patient is comfort care).
5. Adjust medications as needed, such as titrating drips and IV medications according to the patient's vital signs and clinical status.
6. Contact the doctor about necessary changes to drugs that aren't titratable.
7. Give medications as conditions occur, such as Ativan for seizures. (*Oh, the patient has a headache, but the doc hasn't ordered Tylenol? Call the doc, take ten minutes (or longer) to get an order for over-the-counter Tylenol.*) Nausea meds. Anxiety meds. Pre-procedure meds.
8. Obtain, manage, and keep IV access (*the standard is at least one to two IV lines*).
9. If unable to keep IV access, get an order for a central line or midline and assist with line placement as needed.
10. Verify drug compatibilities, knowing what drugs can be given with other drugs—especially IV drugs (*and if you don't, you'd better know exactly where to find this info to be able to administer the medication on time*).
11. Ensure that patients' blood is drawn for the right labs at the right time for the right reasons by the right person.
12. Log in to a computer to check the lab values one to two hours after all lab draws.
13. Replace electrolytes as needed after obtaining replacement protocol orders from the doctor.
14. Report critical or abnormal lab results to the physician and await new orders.

15. Take diabetic patients' blood sugar levels three to four (or more) times during your shift. Cover with insulin injections per protocols.
16. Be able to confidently read radiological test results (like an MRI or CT scan), laboratory results, and any other test results that a patient may go through in the hospital.
17. Interpret lab results and anticipate what is going to be done for the patient regarding any issues that arise.
18. Perform complete head-to-toe assessments at least once a shift and each time there is a change in the patient's status.
19. Take vital signs and interpret them.
20. Know when a patient is about to go downhill and act before something bad happens.
21. Help patients order three meals a day.
22. Ensure that your patients eat those three meals.
23. Make sure patients do not eat if they aren't supposed to.
24. Record and know how much of each meal each patient has eaten and drunk.
25. Keep track of when patients go to the bathroom, both stool and urine, and, in most cases, measure the amount, the color, and the shape.
26. Make sure that patients are comfortable temperature-wise every hour.
27. Make sure that patients are in a comfortable position every one to two hours.
28. Turn patients who are unable to shift their own weight every two hours.
29. Ensure patients have all the things that they need, like their phone, call light, and water.

30. Ensure that no patient ever sits in their own feces or urine for any amount of time.
31. Shower patients who haven't had a shower within the last 48 hours (or whatever the protocol of your facility is).
32. Perform wound care or incision care multiple times per day. (*The surgeon usually only comes the day after surgery; wound care nurses come when able, but they are also drowning in overwork.*)
33. Ensure your patient gets to dialysis and has everything they need before and after.
34. Ensure patients have all the prep that they need for any surgeries or tests that will be performed.
35. Anticipate doctors' needs and have all supplies needed for procedures ready.
36. After a doctor sees your patient, make sure that orders were placed in the computer according to what they told the patient. If they aren't in, contact the doctor to remind them to do so or confirm what the actual plan is.
37. Be in the room while the doctor is there so that you can hear and observe what they're doing and take verbal orders.
38. Remember to place said verbal orders into the computer so the doctor can sign them later, or double-check all orders put in by a doctor to make sure they make sense and were put in correctly.
39. Ensure each patient has been followed up on by each specialty doctor as needed.
40. If no follow-up has been done, page or contact the specialist doctor and request a visit.
41. Make sure all doctors have updated the patient and/or their family about what is going on.

42. Update the patient and/or family if the doctor is unable to, but only within your scope of practice.
43. After the doctor leaves, address patient/family questions about what the doctor said.
44. Update whiteboards (in the patient rooms) with nurse name and phone number, the doctors' names, and the patient's goals.
45. Update and deal with family (*this should be numbers 45–129, but I digress . . .*).
46. Meet all spiritual needs of the patient and family members. (*You could walk from one room with an atheist fighting cancer to another room with a devout pastor with diabetes and liver failure.*)
47. Provide culturally competent care for every possible culture that walks through the doors (for patient and family).
48. Be willing and able to find out about these cultures, religions, ethnicities, and countries of origin on the fly enough to be able to take care of the patient and their family without offending someone or causing an issue.
49. Be able to apologize sufficiently when an accidental error is made that culturally, morally, ethically, medically, or racially offends a patient or their family, no matter who is responsible.
50. Be prepared to apologize to patients or their families when they are upset about something, even if the care provided was correct and no medical error occurred.
51. Manage visitors, and how many, according to the patient's status, and prepare the patient if needed. Deal with the ramifications of upset families.

52. Coordinate with respiratory therapy (RT) to ensure they provide the patient's breathing treatments in a reasonable amount of time.
53. Call RT if the patient's respiratory status is changing.
54. Answer and field phone calls from other departments like laboratory, security, or radiology.
55. Answer and field text messages from other departments.
56. If in a locked unit, manage letting people in and out.
57. Be an IT/tech person by being the first one who has to troubleshoot items in patient rooms like TVs or remotes.
58. Figure out why their bed isn't working correctly and then do something about it if you can't fix it.
59. If drugs are not available from the pharmacy, call them. Keep calling them until the drugs are sent for your use.
60. Not only be aware of, but essentially memorize all your patients' primary diagnoses, medical histories, allergies, and treatment regimens.
61. Be able to answer multiple questions on the fly from doctors or their support personnel at any time.
62. Be able to provide suggestions and requests to the doctors for your patients when appropriate (*because trust me, they ask*).
63. If your patient has COVID or another contagious disease requiring isolation, you need to add onto this gown and glove and masking and suiting up for every single time you step into this patient's room.
64. Charting: documenting all the above in the EMR (electronic medical record).

(Forgive me if I have missed something, the duties of a nurse are so overwhelming that I had literal PTSD typing this list up.)

The amount of charting that a nurse must do is completely crazy. Our employers are now telling us that documentation is the most important part of our job as, without it, they will not get reimbursed and we would not have jobs.

So, our priorities have shifted greatly from being able to take care of patients with very few worries about money, to now having to be obsessed with our wording and verbiage so we get paid. All the correct boxes must be checked, and everything that we did or did not do must be documented for every patient. It is not enough that we did CPR on a patient and had to administer multiple life-saving medications, but we must document to the minute when these were given and how much was given. If there is not a scribe documenting during a "code" in the hospital, this is a major offense and could lead to lawsuits and lack of reimbursement for very expensive hospitalizations and treatments.

Oh, you changed a patient's wound dressing? Nothing can be inferred, so you better document every single thing you did, down to the detail of what you cleaned it with, that you took the old dressing off first, and exactly what the wound looked like when you saw it. Better yet, take a picture of that wound but make sure you document in your note that a picture was taken.

Administered an ordered medication? It's not enough to document that it was given. You also need to record the exact time—usually by scanning the medication and the patient's ID band with your device—the method used (such as by mouth, IV drip, quick IV injection, under the skin, through a feeding tube, or with a skin patch for absorption—called transdermal), and, in many cases, the patient's reaction.

Took someone's glucose level? It's not enough to say you took it and what the result was, you must also document that you cleaned the glucometer machine, the patient's symptoms or lack of them, and how much insulin you gave or why you didn't give any.

Work in the ICU? Better make sure you not only assess the patient every 15 minutes, but that vital signs are being cycled through and taken every 15 minutes and then documented if the patient is critically ill.

Make sure every single time the patient was repositioned, you are documenting that it was done and which side they were left on. Make sure every time you titrate or adjust an IV medication, it is documented (this can be as frequent as every minute!).

A patient refused medication or intervention? Cool. You'd better notify the doctor; in some cases notify the family, notify your nursing supervisor, and document that the patient refused and list all the people you notified and via which route (text/call, etc.). You also need to ensure that later you are documenting if the patient had any adverse effects related to refusing their medication or intervention.

Had a phone conversation with a patient's family member? Better document that shit. Your patient fell? SUPER cool. Now you've gotta assess and document vital signs, neurological checks, and overall clinical status every five minutes for 15 minutes, then every 15 minutes for an hour (or two), and then every hour for twelve hours.

None of this might sound *that* awful until you are taking care of five to seven of such patients at the same time for twelve consecutive hours. The shit never stops; it literally never ends. It is difficult to express the level of exhaustion that a nurse feels.

What the general public doesn't know is that, beyond documentation, nurses are told time and time again that the buck stops with us. That we are the patient's lifeline, and that we must represent them and ensure that no harm comes to them from any other person on our multidisciplinary team, or their family, or any other reason at all. That is a massive amount of pressure that is difficult to understand unless you've experienced it.

Nurses are responsible for not only our own actions, but those of all members of our team, AND for the entire lives of our patients. Plus, we need to be good team members and help our fellow nurses succeed and assist them when needed. Not many people can pull a 400-pound person up in bed alone.

In Part I, you might have noticed how frequently I was chasing people down for help or being chased down by people who need help to do their jobs. I gave advice/suggestions to the doctors, followed up on a medical equipment company's responsibility to get a dying patient home, and had to talk to families on the phone even though a doctor already had. There are days that it feels like no one can do anything without being reminded or guided by me.

Responsibility like that should be way above my pay grade, given what my pay grade is.

What happens if we didn't get enough sleep last night? If our baby was up most of the night and we stayed up with them? What about a sick child, family member, or parent who lives with us? What about if we are fighting with our spouse and are distracted mentally? What if our pet is sick or high maintenance? What if WE don't feel well? What if we are on our sixth twelve-hour shift in a row and just don't have the same brain capacity as we did on day one?

Hopefully nothing happens . . . but there is a chance that some balls may be dropped during a shift or–God forbid–someone's life affected negatively forever.

Healthcare workers are expected to shoulder these enormous physical, mental, and emotional burdens at work, and just be able to handle those *plus* the stressors of normal life without any problems. We are expected to just "figure it out" and make sure we are not only providing good clinical care, but meeting all the "wants" of the patient and their families (like ice-cold water and a flat-screen TV).

How can we continue shouldering this massive workload?

The answer is: we can't. Nurses are looking for any other type of nursing job except bedside. I belong to several nursing groups on social media, and they are full to the brim with nurses who are sick of bedside nursing and want out. The daily to-do list of a nurse cannot continue to be added to without more help and support being provided.

During my management days in home health, I felt like I was asking more from my nurses on a weekly basis. I would have to bring them in, have a meeting, and ask them to do more. Keep track of more. Document more. Put more and more on their plates as the days went by. After a while, it gets exhausting. I never had to ask the physical therapist to make sure the nurse was doing their job, but I certainly had to ask the nurse to make sure the therapist was doing their job (and document it).

It's worse in a hospital. The amount of shit that a nurse must keep track of for every one of their patients is overwhelming. In the story I shared in Part I, I was already a veteran by that point; doing it long enough that remembering all the details and requirements had become habit. But there were still many times a day I had to re-route myself back to my own role because I was juggling so many balls and having to keep track of so many things, as well as support coworkers.

Imagine having a sick parent. I'm sure many of you have had to handle this. Many of you will in the future.

Imagine your parent is sick and weak and lives with you, relying on you 24/7 to ensure they are safe and have everything they need—food, water, shelter, comfort, and medications. You are responsible for keeping track of them and providing transportation to and from any appointments they have.

You must know what went on during those appointments, write down the results and any new medications, treatments, or interventions needed, and make sure your parent is taken care of during all of this. You need to answer them every time they call for you.

You must update your other family members daily as to how your parent is, what has changed, and how much they are eating at every meal. If they are incontinent, you are responsible for cleaning them up and getting them changed every single time (that's at least four to six times a day and throughout the night). You need to make sure they stay hydrated and fed, and control their pain by giving them medications every four to six hours (or more often).

You must help them get dressed in the morning and ready for bed at night. You must make sure they get their shower, during which you do about 75% of the work because they are too weak to do it themselves. You must comfort them, be there for them, and advocate for them with their doctors, therapists, and other specialists.

Finally, you need to get them anything they need or want in a timely manner—and do so politely every single time—because you will not get paid any money if you do not have good customer service skills toward them.

Exhausting, eh?

Now imagine adding five more people to the mix that you must do the same for. And you're not even related to them. Yeah . . . and none of these things I just mentioned even scratch the surface of the medical skills that are put into play as a nurse, like monitoring vitals, labs, IV meds, etc.

I have had several nursing students—before they even graduate—tell me they were burnt out, have lost interest in their career, or have been thinking about changing careers already. That is so sad. When I came out of nursing school, I was full of piss and vinegar and ready to save the world with my big brain and tough feet.

This field used to be exciting, a great career, a good and reliable way to make money for your family but also enjoy your life with four days off a week. Patients were generally respectable and grateful.

It has now become a tumultuous, exhausting, and frustrating job where it feels like you are constantly drowning and can never catch up. There's an ongoing joke that healthcare workers are in an abusive relationship with their jobs. It's funny, but also not funny at all.

I have also watched doctors—having gone through med school and residency—immediately want to, or actually, quit.

Now, let me pause and say this. I also know many healthcare workers who still very much love what they do. Their reward is making a difference and taking care of people in their darkest hour. They feel fulfilled and good about themselves and their careers, for the most part.

One of my coworkers, who's been a nurse for 15 years, says what keeps her going are the few patients each year who are genuinely grateful—those whose lives she was truly able to save and make a difference in. She said, "I have a thank-you note from a patient hanging on my mirror in my bathroom that helps me get out of bed and continue to do this day in and day out."

Sometimes it doesn't take much to keep a healthcare provider going. We can take care of 100 shitty people who are rude and abusive but then take care of one who buys us a cup of coffee and writes a note, and we are re-invigorated to continue to take care of people and do what we are called to do.

(Technically, this how the abuse cycle in a relationship works, hence the ongoing joke.)

It takes a very special person to be able to do what a nurse, doctor, or CNA (or any healthcare professional) does on a daily basis, and usually those who don't fit the mold quit and move to a different career within a short amount of time. But even those who claim to still love what they do are still very aware of the challenges of the profession. They see that the healthcare system in America is failing healthcare workers and patients alike.

They too can see the writing on the wall.

I wish we could go back to the days when we only had to take care of the patient. In other words, I wish we could treat their disease process, stabilize them, do some education, and then discharge them. If so, we would likely be able to keep up with the demands of current healthcare. But in today's world, on top of being their nurse, we are expected to be hotel managers, waitresses, therapists, personal attendants, and personal advocates for each and every one of our patients. This is asking a hell of a lot from one human being.

Let's put this in perspective. Back in the 1950s, a nurse took care of 50 patients by themselves. Their list of daily duties included the following:[1]

1. Daily sweep and mop of the floors of your ward.
2. Dust furniture and windowsills.
3. Maintain an even temperature in your ward by bringing in coal each day.
4. Fill kerosene lamps, trim wicks, and clean chimneys. Wash windows once weekly.
5. Ensure your handwriting is legible for the doctor to read in your nurses' notes.

6. Monitor the patient's temperature and overall status throughout the day and report to the doctor any changes in condition.
7. When a doctor enters the ward, the nurse will stand, hand the patient's chart directly to the doctor, offer her chair, and ensure he is comfortable while he works.

That's it. Nurses did basically no medical care without specific request from the doctor. No medications were given without a doctor being right there. Nurses didn't even take blood pressures or use stethoscopes!

Ahh . . . what a life they led. So easy and simple. It was even MORE simple in Florence Nightingale's time in the 1800s. Compared to the insane amount of shit on a present-day nurse's plate, this list is a literal walk in the park. Good ole Florence would have a damn heart attack if she walked into a modern-day hospital and saw the workload of a nurse. Florence paid amazing attention to detail when it came to infection control and bless her for that . . . but Florence don't know shit when it comes to being a nurse nowadays.

Before the transition to a performance-based reimbursement system with Medicare and Medicaid, the most important thing about a patient's hospital stay was that they got better. Now, the most important thing is that they got their lunch on time and their TV worked appropriately.

I've already spoken about how this has changed the face of healthcare in a very negative way. It has also increased the workload of a nurse tenfold. Most patients now act entitled, a little spoiled, and as if all healthcare workers are there to serve them; not use our clinical knowledge to fix them. I mean, the NERVE of us if we prioritize doing CPR on a patient over getting Bobby an ice water in room 314.

Performance-based reimbursement is where the good ole days ended.

Medicare's website, CMS.gov, has a very short explanation about performance-based reimbursement. They call them *value-based programs*. They state, "Our value-based programs are important because they're helping us move toward paying providers based on the quality, rather than the quantity of care they give patients."[2]

Okay, makes sense. I understand that it's better to make sure we slow down a bit, set patients up for success, and make sure we have good outcomes. I also understand that some hospitals in the past have rushed patients through the steps of care to get them out the door to make room for the next patient to make more money and have more insurance claims. I hear the concerns that hospitals are all about the dollar and not about the patient.

In fact, I can directly see the results of that mentality across our nation. But I'm not sure that the value-based programs are the solution. In fact, I think that these programs are hindering our ability to provide great medical care by making us terrified of not getting paid. It misaligns our priorities as a medical system away from caring and healing, to pleasing patients and catering to them.

The biggest issue by far with these programs is that this culture has made patients and their families more entitled. It drastically increases the workload of healthcare workers because now we are not only in charge of making patients better, we are also driven to please them in every aspect while they are under our care. This shift in mentality—from treating people as patients ("We want to take care of you and make you better") to treating them as consumers ("What can we do for you?")—is one of the main roots of the problems in healthcare.

I understand that some doctors in private practices have

increased their incomes because of these programs, but the truth is these were the top performers anyway. I want them to continue to be rewarded for their exceptional care, but the program is inherently flawed because it does not *actually* improve the poor performers.

Pay for performance programs add to the proverbial plates of nurses and healthcare workers, which are already overflowing, with no scientific data backing their appropriateness, success, or failure. It is shocking to me the amount of shit a nurse must do daily just to maintain their patients; it is exhausting both mentally and physically. Never mind all the additional things that continue to be piled onto nurses' plates without regard to the things falling off the back of it.

When is enough, enough?

We are burnt out before we are even out of school and we don't want to do this anymore. ICUs, ERs, and hospitals in general are overflowing with patients who are so sick that we cannot keep up with them.

We are drowning under the burden the American healthcare system places on us by overloading us at every turn to save a buck.

CHAPTER 5

THE COST OF CARE

THE TRUE VALUE OF NURSES IN A BROKEN SYSTEM

WE'VE all seen the ads, right?

> Hiiiii!!! I'm MONICA and I USED to be a BEDSIDE NURSE! 😊 But NOW I am a millionaire because bedside nursing SUCKS 😷🤮💩🤢🤕😭 and I decided to become an entrepreneur and used my NURSING KNOWLEDGE🧠 to design sparkly coffee mugs on Etsy! ☕NOW I can day drink 🍸 💅 and basically print my own money 🤑 !!!

They are all over social media. Like, thanks, Monica, but shut the hell up. There are also legit RNs who have taken their nursing license and turned it into some crazy seven-figure income doing something nuts like *teaching nurses how to take care of themselves.*

I mean, good for y'all.

According to the Bureau of Labor Statistics, the average RN in America makes about $86,000 per year.[1] There are low-paying states, such as Mississippi, Alabama, and West Virginia, where average pay is around $65,000 per year (GASP).[2] Then there are the high-paying states such as California, Hawaii, and Massachusetts, that pay over $105,000 per year.[3]

Remember, "average" means counting everyone at every level of the career—not what nurses make right out of school.

A study in March 2024 by smartasset.com reported that, to live comfortably as a *single* person in America, you need to make an average of $96,500 a year.[4] They define "living comfortably" as being able to pay your bills, feed yourself, pay off debt, and invest for the future. While that's crazy to think about, it's terrifying to see that they also state that a family of four (two adults and two children) requires $235,000 a year to NOT live paycheck to paycheck.

RNs are objectively underpaid in two ways. First, they are paid less than it costs to live in this nation. This is a statistically and personally significant problem, as we all need to pay our bills and be able to afford basic necessities such as food and shelter. Second, the responsibility level placed on nurses is astronomical.

The complexity of patient care, the emotional and mental burden of caring for the sick, constantly working understaffed, legal and ethical expectations, our role in coordinating care, the length of our shifts, and the physical demands of the job are too much for one person to endure. These stressors, combined with a compensation rate that doesn't even meet the cost of living means we feel extremely undervalued. Despite frequently being described as the "backbone" of the healthcare system—and indeed we are, we do not have the safe working conditions or pay to show for it.

How about this? How about we make bedside nursing less terrible so that we don't have to design some arbitrary way to make an actual living that doesn't suck the literal souls out of us?

I'm not saying all nurses should be paid a million bucks by

their employers. What I'm saying is that, if we were able to make bedside nursing a little less abusive, a little less draining, a little less . . . *shitty* . . . then maybe we would be able to continually staff happy, fulfilled, and skilled nurses.

Instead, we keep dumping more and more on nurses' plates, making them responsible for what should be instantly recognized as a completely unreasonable number of things to expect one human to do. And *then* we pay them a wage that is nowhere near comparable to the type of work and responsibility level.

The working-class American is beginning to stand taller. We are starting to demand that we are paid attention to. These enormous companies with astronomical profit margins need to disseminate more of that profit to their frontline people—especially in healthcare. I'd like the CEO of a large hospital to follow a CNA around and do *their* job. Like actually wipe a person's ass and get screamed at, hit, and demeaned while doing it. And then go home with a CNA's paycheck and see how they like life. Your $500k+ salary to go to meetings and "represent" this hospital seems like a joke compared to the importance of a CNA. I would LOVE to see an *Undercover Boss* with a hospital administrator pretending to be a nurse, CNA or doc.

If nurses and other support staff of a hospital do not start being protected and paid a livable wage, there will be very few left to do the job. According to Medscape.com, around 900,000 nurses are planning to leave the profession by 2027.[5] That's about a fifth of ALL nurses in America!

Let's be conservative and say that 15 percent of the nursing workforce leaves the profession altogether. If a hospital floor takes twelve nurses to run at full staffing, that means two to three of them have quit. Therefore, the nine nurses left have to pick up one to three extra patients each. If a nurse is already starting with six patients, that means they are taking care of up to NINE sick patients at a time.

Those ratios are not sustainable for safe and excellent care. It's either this, or the hospital has to block off beds, which results in decreased profits. I'm sure you can imagine how often that happens.

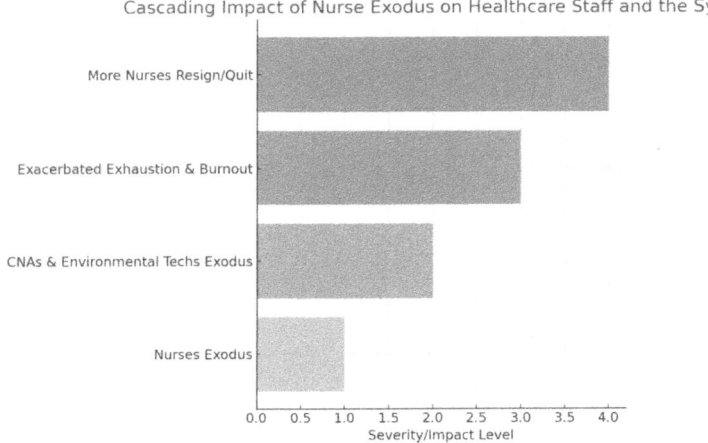

With the exodus of nurses, there will be an even more severe exodus of CNAs and environmental techs, which will exacerbate the exhaustion and burnout of the nurses who are left, which in turn will cause more nurses to resign or quit the profession altogether. Nurses are starting to come out of school wanting to become Botox injectors instead of floor nurses. Can't blame them.

Medscape.com estimates that around 33% of new grad nurses quit the profession entirely with two years of graduation because of burn out and working conditions.[6] The simple fact that hospitals are either unwilling or unable (it doesn't matter which) to pay their support personnel a livable wage is going to change the face of American healthcare as we know it. It already has.

I say it doesn't matter whether a hospital is unwilling or unable to pay a living wage because it is not the employee's problem that hospitals cannot afford to run correctly. There has to be a solution to them being able to pay us a comparable livable wage.

The low pay fails to compensate by far for the 80% of nurses that report abuse of some kind in the workplace, combined with the amount of responsibility on our shoulders.[7] If this continues, hospitals are in for a world of hurt, and I would say they need to start making some serious changes.

As a patient, what you will start seeing is hospital stays that are hospital "stays," meaning you will not be getting your ice water as soon as you've requested it. Your TV volume may be stuck on the highest setting for the entirety of your stay or may not work at all. You won't be getting your pain pill on time, and you most likely will end up peeing your bed because answering call bells will be impossible. Your breakfast tray has been sitting there for an hour? That sucks.

Having someone available to sit down with you for 45 minutes and educate you on your new diagnosis, new medications, treatments, and how to manage all of this on your own at home will also basically not exist. You will be on your own. Google it. Get your own medical degree because ours will be on our wall while, as Monica as showed us, we use our Cricut machines to make glittery mugs while we day drink and listen to gangster rap.

Every single person should be fighting to get healthcare workers an average livable wage comparable with current inflation. If the government can bail out BILLIONS or TRILLIONS of dollars when a bunch of banks go under, they can certainly do the same for hospitals post-global pandemic and moving into the future. There are hospital conglomerates all over the United States that absolutely have the resources to pay their workers better.

How do I know? Because of travelers.

Contracted employees/nurses (or "travelers") make about twice the amount of money a normal, staffed, full-time employee makes. If a hospital is understaffed with nurses, they will reach out to a hiring agency. This agency charges a much higher hourly wage for this person to come in and work. Let's say that hourly wage is $120. Instead of paying about $40 for a staff RN, the hospital pays this agency $120 an hour for their nurse to come and work three to four twelve-hour shifts for 13 weeks, or so.

These contracted nurses make on average about $20 of that $120 an hour, plus they get a tax-free housing stipend of at least $1,400 a week that comes out of that higher hourly wage as well. So even if their hourly wage is technically less than the $40 they'd make on staff, that tax-free living stipend pushes them up into the double or triple cost space for the facility itself.

Now, prior to COVID, travel nurses were mostly rare. In a good, reputable, stable facility, there would be one traveler for every ten full-time employees, or maybe even less. It is almost reversed now.

From what I've heard, travel nurses now make up as much as 70% of the staff in some of these same reputable, stable facilities. COVID showed nurses that all they had to do was sign up with a travel company, and they could make as much in 13 weeks as they previously did in 6 months or more. And let's not get into the mid-COVID bonus money these agencies were paying nurses. Normal RNs with no advanced degrees were getting paid $150 an hour plus bonuses and stipends on contracts in high-demand places across America.

This was equating to $6,000 or more *take-home pay* PER WEEK! Nurses were taking two 13-week contracts and literally changing their lives. No more school debt. Car paid off. Credit cards paid off completely. Massive chunk of money in savings.

Now that COVID is over, the travel nurse rates are getting back to normal, but the number of travel nurses is still high. It's much easier mentally to be a travel nurse because you are getting paid more and you really do not need to get mentally invested in the hospital you are working in. Have a crappy manager? Don't take another assignment there! Benefits not great at that facility? You don't care because you don't need them! Another fantastic benefit of travel nursing is that the wages are so good, you can schedule weeks off at a time in between contracts, if you manage your money well. This is time to reflect, recharge, and take care of yourself before diving into another stressful 13 weeks.

The point is this. If hospitals can afford to outsource even 20 percent of their staff to expensive staffing agencies—paying rates two to three times higher than what they give full-time employees—for months on end without going bankrupt, then why can't they offer salaries that align with today's cost of living?

The answer is, in most cases, they CAN. We are not asking for $100,000 raises here. But look at the plate that I was talking about in the previous chapter—we should have a good base pay for nurses that matches that level of responsibility. Yeah, I know that number seems like a lot when you add up the hundreds of employees that would need this raise, but . . . so? What costs more: giving these raises, or people dying because medical care is poor or not available?

Most hospitals—especially rural ones—are operating with a very slim profit margin. If hospitals are going to end up closing anyhow, we might as well hurry this along, close the ones that aren't going to make it, and give us the choice of which facility to work for that can afford to stay open and pay well.

If hospitals across America are going bankrupt right now because of the increased costs associated with contracted employees, residual effects of COVID, inflation costs of supplies and medications, and decreased reimbursement rates because of insurance companies, then I cannot imagine what is going to happen when the shit ACTUALLY hits the fan. We think we are in the recovery phase from this pandemic, and I really pray that we are. But I have a feeling we have only just scratched the surface of an arterially bleeding wound that is going to be very difficult to recover from across the healthcare continuum.

Nurses and other healthcare professionals who lived through and survived the three-year COVID shitstorm will never be the same.

When I asked ChatGPT if it thought that hospitals could pay RNs more, it said, "Hospitals could likely pay RNs more, but the situation is complex and depends on various factors."

The factors it mentions are the ones I have already talked about, including the reliance on travel nurses, reimbursement rates, overall cost of healthcare (such as equipment), and administrative overhead and burden. I have seen firsthand the pressure that administrative burden puts on healthcare facilities, and it is paralyzing. The United States is the only country in the world that places this type of burden on its healthcare system.

According to my friend ChatGPT, up to 35% of a hospital's employees on average are administrative. These include IT, billing/coding for reimbursement, human resources, marketing, upper management, middle management, environmental services/janitorial staff, and administrative assistants or support staff.

America has bogged down its healthcare system with such a fractionated and confusing billing/reimbursement process that these facilities have had to create multiple departments just to get paid. Another part of this issue is all the regulations put in place on *every single aspect* of the delivery of healthcare. This requires people and positions to ensure that all regulations are being followed in each department (hence the creation of middle management). The transition to value-based care models has added even more administrative burden because we now have to hire people to keep track of and report on all the new data from patient satisfaction surveys.

Let's not even mention the salaries of these C-suite people (in hospitals especially). The salaries of hospital executives in this country are among the highest *in the entire world*, adding significantly to the overhead burden of these facilities.[8] Imagine if we lived in a country where a CEO of a hospital wasn't paid one dollar more a year than their lowest paid doctor. (No offense, but I think that a surgeon should make more than a hospital CEO.)

All of this to say: We could make small but significant changes to the system to create room in the budget to pay nurses more, giving us more incentive to stay in the profession. Although pay is not the only piece to this puzzle, it is a very large one.

Nurses are the lifeblood of the healthcare system, shouldering unimaginable levels of responsibility and stress. We are the ones catching critical errors, coordinating care, advocating for patients, and providing physical, emotional, and mental support—all while enduring the immense pressure of understaffed shifts and overwhelming workloads. And yet, our compensation rarely reflects the weight of these responsibilities. Being expected to manage the lives of others while struggling to afford the cost of our own is not just insulting and unjust—it's unsustainable.

Livable wages that account for the cost of living and the magnitude of our responsibilities are the bare minimum. Feeling valued isn't just about paychecks; it's about knowing that the system sees and respects the sacrifices we make every single day. Without this fundamental shift, the nursing profession will continue to hemorrhage talent, leaving behind a fragile healthcare system unable to meet the needs of those it serves.

The truth is, when nurses are supported—through fair pay, safe working conditions, and genuine appreciation—patients thrive, and the entire system benefits.

CHAPTER 6

THE OVERWORKED, UNDERPAID, AND INDISPENSABLE CNAS

FOR THOSE OF you who do not know what a CNA is, let me introduce you to the backbone of a hospital.

CNAs, or Certified Nurse Assistants, are licensed personnel who help you with personal care tasks when you're sick. These are the angels who help you to the bathroom, clean you up when you're incontinent, give you a bed bath, get you into the shower, set up your meals, feed you, help you brush your teeth, brush your hair (the good ones even braid it because they know how bad bed head can get), take your vital signs, and report anything abnormal to the nurse. They are in your room the most often, have the most direct contact with you during your hospitalization, and are commonly the number one voice for you.

Nurses who do not respect and revere their CNAs are assholes.

In my opinion, being a CNA is one of the hardest jobs on planet earth. Their job is physically, emotionally, and mentally exhausting. They are most often the first line of defense and therefore most abused when patients get out of control. They are the ones in the rooms getting berated and yelled at first; they are the ones dealing with literal and metaphorical shit all day. It is a true calling to do this line of work, day in and day out. I've witnessed the most beautiful, sweetest interactions between CNAs and their patients.

Can you imagine giving a shower to someone who can only do 50% of the work? Not only are you holding them up, but you're trying to get all their folds and crevices clean while trying not to get soaked yourself. Or how about a bed bath where you are doing 100% of the work? Or dealing with feces and urine all day every day? Or keeping track of like ten to 20 patients and their well-being, toileting, and statuses?

When I first became a nurse, the first thing I noticed was that CNAs never sit down. They don't have the amount of charting that RNs do, so they are up and on their feet literally all day long. They are the ones answering all the call bells 90% of the time. They are constantly running from one end of the unit to the other.

To care for people in the most intimate way for years and years on end takes its toll. You must be excellent at compartmentalizing and be able to (at least mostly) leave work at work. Being a CNA is a different world to being a nurse. Nurses are more on the assessment, critical thinking, monitoring, and management side of a patient's healthcare team. CNAs are on the compassionate, personal, down-and-dirty level. Not that nurses aren't compassionate—and not that we don't get down and dirty within a patient's life with them—but it's just not to the same degree that CNAs do.

But let's step back briefly and look at the real life of a CNA.

When I first became a nurse 15 years ago, I worked at a long-term care facility, and there were several career CNAs on my floor. There were at least five who had been CNAs for over

20 years (which is *mind-blowing* to me). Now though? I bet less than ten percent of all CNAs in America have been one for over 20 years. It is the exception rather than the rule now. A job as a CNA is now a steppingstone to becoming a nurse, or an interim job that people do for a while until they can find something better. But honestly, who can blame them? The average CNA in America is paid $18 an hour.[1] That's about $37,000 per year.

For the amount of work that these people do, this wage is a disgrace.

To give this some context, McDonald's advertises on Indeed.com that their lowest level crew members make $14.81 an hour in my home state of Colorado.[2] According to Ziprecruiter.com, CNAs in Colorado are paid an average of $19.15 an hour.[3] A starting job at McDonald's deserves respect but it requires no degree, no certificate, no specialty training, and no one's lives in your hands. CNAs making only $10k a year more than an entry-level McDonald's worker is astounding to me. No wonder no one does this for a career anymore.

Another challenge facing CNAs is hours being cut. Hospitals across the nation have deemed CNAs to be essentially a "luxury item" on their staff, and they've decided that technically nurses should be able to just pick up all the CNAs' responsibilities and do them on top of their existing workloads. My hospital currently has one CNA for 20 ICU patients, and no unit secretary.*

That means that the one solitary CNA that we have on our entire floor is responsible for all the showers and baths,

---

* A unit secretary is the person who directs guests, answers the phone, gets messages to the correct person, and overall has a hold on what's going on in the unit answering the majority of call lights, answering the door for guests (our ICU is a locked unit), answering the phone, and helping any nurses with any other task needed, including but not at all limited to getting patients on and off a bedpan, pulling a patient up in bed, turning a patient, feeding a patient, getting water, filling ice packs, taking vitals, bringing supplies into a room, reorienting a patient to prevent them from falling, etc.

That CNA's butt does not touch the chair all day long.

CNAs are *not luxury items*. The workload of nurses and all our responsibilities is only made remotely possible because of what CNAs do. In the ICU, we nurses typically only have two patients each, so doing our own patient care is a lot more realistic than on other floors. If there were no CNAs on a medical-surgical floor, I cannot even imagine the chaos that would ensue.

Patients would fall. They would decompensate and get very sick. Hygiene would plummet, and therefore infections would increase. I bet dehydration would also increase. Nurses simply cannot do everything that they are required to do *in addition* to the job of a CNA. It's scary to think what would happen if CNAs were to start quitting for higher-paying jobs with less responsibility and fuckery. Oh wait . . . that's already happening.

We need to start paying attention to retaining CNAs in hospitals and long-term care facilities because this will have a domino effect, as a lack of CNAs will make nurses eventually quit, too. Having the load that a nurse has with no backup at all is impossible.

The CNAs that I know are almost all nursing students working one to two days a week at the most, just using the role to gain experience and a little bit of money while at school. Although this is a wonderful plan for them, and they contribute in the role, it is difficult for patients and means a lack of continuity of care that is necessary for positive outcomes.

Back in the good old days, a patient would have the same CNA for three to five days in a row. This did wonders to help patients develop a sense of trust and comradery with the people taking care of their most intimate needs. I've seen some patients just absolutely thrive in the presence of a CNA that they jive well with. I've also seen many patients experience poor outcomes because they have no trust or relationship with the constant influx of new people.

There are many things that set a patient up for success when they are hospitalized, placed in a long-term care facility, or at a rehab center. In my opinion, CNAs are at the top of that list. If you have a wonderful CNA who is on their game, taking great care of their patients, the outcomes will reflect this. Of course, on the contrary, if you have a CNA that hides all day and slacks off, you can totally see that too.

There is a long-term acute care (LTAC) facility that sometimes transfers patients to us that has very subpar CNA staff. I am not sure if this is because of the facility itself keeping them constantly understaffed, or if the actual workers themselves are the problem, but it is shameful. We get referred patients into the ICU from this facility with very severe pressure injuries (wounds) and actual *layers* of dead skin cells, sweat, and dirt on them. They haven't been bathed in weeks. And most of these patients are paraplegics, quadriplegics, or are otherwise severely physically handicapped and are permanently on life support. I have no idea how this facility is still open.

There's another long-term care facility that I get patients from whose patients are beautifully taken care of. You can just tell that they have stellar CNAs and staff there. The patients are clean, with few if any wounds, and you can tell they are well managed.

No one should have layers of dirt on them, that's literal neglect and is inhumane. But if a facility isn't willing to staff enough CNAs to support the needs of their patients, there is little that can be done with minimal resources. If I was a CNA at a facility like that LTAC, I would quit before you could say "this is a fucking joke." There's no way I would be able to tolerate working under those conditions. I would also report them to the state on my way out the door.

CNAs are the lifeblood of any good medical floor, facility, or agency. They are the hands that bathe, the feet that run, and the hearts that uplift those in their most vulnerable moments. Yet, despite their vital role, CNAs are chronically underpaid, overworked, and undervalued. Their work is not just physically exhausting; it demands a level of compassion and emotional resilience that few other jobs require.

This is a systemic issue that we cannot ignore. When CNAs are unsupported—when they are stretched too thin, dismissed as "luxuries," or paid wages that barely sustain them —it sets off a chain reaction. Patient care suffers, nurses burn out, and the entire healthcare system begins to suffer. Without CNAs, hospitals, long-term care facilities, and rehabilitation centers cannot function safely or well. These dedicated individuals deserve more than gratitude; they deserve fair pay, adequate staffing, and a workplace that values their well-being as much as the patients they care for.

Without CNAs?

Oh man. We would be so screwed.

CHAPTER 7

FROM HEALERS TO HUSTLERS
THE BURDEN ON MODERN DOCTORS

IT MAY COME as no surprise to hear that doctors are feeling the same way as nurses and CNAs.

They are overwhelmed. They are in such a litigious environment now that many doctors have told me that they unwillingly participate in "defensive medicine," which is where they order tests, scans, or interventions purely to cover their own asses in case a patient or family member sues.[1]

They openly admit to requesting interventions, not because a patient needs them, but because, if they don't, it could look bad on them, or they risk not getting paid. They complain that much of their job has been about CYA (cover your ass) rather than truly patient-centered care. They are exhausted from all the regulations that are being placed on their shoulders. In so many cases, doctors are not even able to fully be doctors. They used to be the root of all of healthcare—they used to make all the calls, prescribe anything that was needed, and be where the buck stops. Their plates are also incredibly full.

Doctors must remember all the laws, all the regulations, and all their moral and ethical obligations as healthcare providers. Not to mention all the clinical stuff that they need to remember about patients' minds, bodies, medications, medication interactions, medication side effects, procedures, tests, and lab work. They need to make decisions on a dime—usually with little to no prep time or notice—and it could literally mean life or death for a patient. It is not enough that a doctor knows the results of something, they have to act on it within a reasonable time frame. And when you have many patients under your care, this can become incredibly overwhelming. This is why the good ones heavily rely on their nurses—none of us can do this alone.

Becoming a doctor is *hard*. I mean, becoming a GOOD doctor is hard. There are plenty of people who graduate from medical school and become residents that have no business being doctors. They get into it for the money, because of parental pressure, or for the perceived glamour, fame, and reverence, but are then usually very disappointed.

If I'm in a room with ten doctors, I can tell immediately which ones are in it because being a healer is in their heart and soul versus those doing it for the wrong reasons. When I approach a resident and tell them something is wrong with my patient, but they continue to sit at their computer, typing in nonsensical orders having not even physically assessed the patient, I quickly realize they are not docs in their souls.

The ones who immediately jump up, listen closely to what I'm telling them, and work together with me at bedside as a team, on the other hand, I know are in it for the right reasons.

If you become a doctor for the wrong reasons, countless people suffer. Not only do your coworkers probably hate working with you, but your patients suffer because you feel entitled and as if you know better than them. Granted, you are the medical professional that everyone looks to in the event of shit hitting the fan, so you'd better know more than them!

However, the reality is bedside manner is more important than perfect memorization of anatomy and physiology. If a patient doesn't trust you, feels degraded or shamed by you, or can't understand you when you talk to them, what is the point?

Did you know that doctors go to school, are consistently tested with boards and exams, have ongoing clinicals, internships, residencies, and fellowships for up to (and sometimes more than) 15 YEARS?! So even if you know right out of high school that's what you want to do, and you go through undergrad, get accepted to med school and graduate, then go through residency and likely fellowship for specializing, you are about 35 years old by the time you're a full-fledged attending physician. That's some dedication!

Normally by 35, most people have around ten years of experience in their field after obtaining a four-year degree. But doctors really aren't considered "experienced" until at least their fellowship year. So, by 35, they are for all intents and purposes, still beginners with only three to four years' experience.

Did you also know that resident docs (those who have graduated medical school and are now baby doctors) in America only get paid an average of $60,000? That's literally less than or equal to nurses, depending on what state you're in.

Where I work, the resident ICU rotation is *brutal*. They are required to work six twelve-hour shifts a week for the entire month that they are assigned. These are the sickest patients in the hospital; the neediest, the scariest, and the most fragile. Residents walk around my unit with wide, terrified eyes most of the time. And get paid pennies for it. It's criminal to be honest. It's definitely not glamorous.

These docs have dead eyes, fall asleep sitting up, lose the ability to form proper sentences from exhaustion, and yet are expected to perform at the top of their game at all times. For $30 an hour. I just can't even.

After residency, docs have a couple of choices: they can either go directly into practice and be a private practice/clinic doc/hospitalist, or they can go into fellowship to work towards a subspecialty.

Fellowship means an average of three to five more years of "school," where you are still having to take board exams and work full time. You have more clout and generally more knowledge as a fellow and have residents under your care. Once you qualify as a fellow, you make an average of $80,000 a year in the US, which is better than a resident, but not by much.

I find that fellows are almost always easier to work with than residents because they have enough experience to be confident, but also because they generally love the specialty they are in. It's still not glamorous; these docs rarely see their families (if they have one), they eat hospital food more than any other type of food, and they breathe hospital air WAY more than they do fresh air.

Ironically, but unsurprisingly, they are generally not very healthy people themselves.

Nowadays people Google their symptoms and often attempt to direct their care and interventions with this "knowledge." It's honestly not the Googling that is the problem—if you have a health concern, you *should* be trying to educate yourself on it! No, it's the attitude that accompanies it. People act as if they are smarter than their doctors.

For example, my dad was suffering from debilitating headaches for several months. He would have to pull over his car if he was driving, he would have to go into a dark room, sometimes for hours, to get himself through them. He went to several doctors, all of whom diagnosed him with migraines and sent him on his way. He was given migraine meds that didn't touch his pain. My mom started Googling his symptoms, and during his next appointment, she asked the docs if what he was suffering from was cluster migraines, a debilitating, very severe type of headache. They took this into consideration and eventually, this is what he was diagnosed with.

Even though my parents got frustrated with the whole process, the fact that the docs listened to her and took what she said into consideration resulted in a positive outcome. My dad got the treatment he needed, and he no longer suffers from them.

But throughout this ordeal, my mom remained professional. She was not name-calling the docs, she was not overly demanding. She was just confident in the research that she had done and stated the facts respectfully and knowledgeably. One thing that people tend not to understand is that doctors do not have time to Google and research every patient's symptoms for hours each day. They hardly have enough time to do basic chart reviews on their patients before seeing them.

In fact, this is one of the number one complaints I hear from doctors at all levels, from intern to attending: the lack of time to be able to do a proper chart review. They say that, to do a thorough chart review for all their patients, they need to work much later than they should have to. The number of patients crammed into their days makes it virtually impossible to do even a basic one, never mind a thorough one that could allow them to catch something important. This time crunch means doctors can only focus on small details of a patient's situation, rather than being able to care for their overall health and wellbeing.

In our ICU, patients are more-or-less evenly distributed among the residents. As the "baby" doctors, they get around four to seven patients each (although it's more like ten to 15 on a med-surg ward). The single fellow on the floor, however, is responsible for all 20 patients in the ICU. He or she has all the residents working underneath them, which helps with the busywork of charting, but think about the mental load of this. This doctor must oversee 20 critically ill patients, all of their procedures and totality of their healthcare, *and also* train newbie docs on the ins and outs of critical care, specialty procedures, patient care in general, and being a doctor.

Whoa.

I knew a doctor, several years ago, who decided to go into concierge medicine for this exact reason.* He had been a doctor for around two decades, and he could not handle the herding of patients like cattle into and out of his office. He told me that he was instructed to see one patient every nine to twelve minutes and was not allowed to go over that time.

The clinic he worked for would only allow *one* patient complaint per visit. So, if you had four issues you had questions on and things the doctor needed to address, you had to make separate appointments for each—and of course be charged accordingly.

He said that it was literally impossible for him to truly chart review patients, and he felt like it was causing him to miss things, misdiagnose people, and cause patients harm and suffering. He hated it. He was super stressed out. He couldn't get to know his patients, he had no idea what their home life was like (which can greatly impact a patient's healthcare), and he couldn't take his time to do what he really loved.

So, he opened his own concierge doctor business. He went into private practice with cash-only payments. He charges a monthly fee for people to "belong" to his practice. He will

---

* A concierge doctor is a primary care physician who offers personalized medical care to patients in exchange for a membership or retainer fee, usually paid annually or monthly.

always answer his phone for you or will call back shortly when he's able to. Most days, he can get you an appointment the same day or will make a home visit to you at the end of his business day, if needed.

Your appointment time with him as your doctor is about three to four times as long as one in a typical clinic. He knows all your kids' names. He knows details about your life that affect your healthcare. He knows *why* you suffer from depression and anxiety, not just *that* you are diagnosed with them. He is much happier, more fulfilled, and makes just as much if not more money than when he was billing insurance companies for his service.

Most importantly, there's a huge difference in patient care. He is truly able to change patients' lives.

But for most doctors, no matter what your specialty is, being a doctor is exhausting. The way that insurance works nowadays, doctors are pressured to be more concerned with a patient's coverage than their actual care.

Because here's the deal. If your doc prescribes you a medication that is the most beneficial for your situation, but your insurance doesn't cover it, you are unlikely to be able to afford it for long-term treatments. Therefore, your physician has to dig around for subpar interventions or "approved" medications to treat you so that your insurance pays for it.

I was watching a video the other day of a doctor talking about exactly this. He said that the fact that he had to be as careful as he does with insurance coverage for patient treatments is incredibly detrimental to their well-being and health. He has had to become an expert on insurance coverage, which has taken away from his actual clinical care of patients. It's ridiculous the hoops he has to jump through to just treat his patients.

He gives an example and states that, if he is following a

patient who has a tumor and needs an MRI to have it properly diagnosed and assessed, he will order it, but insurance will deny the claim. He will call and say, "This patient needs an MRI, we have suspicion of cancer and need it diagnosed."

Insurance will come back and say, "Did you order a CT scan first?" and he will say, "No, they don't need a CT scan, they need an MRI."

He will continue to argue with them back and forth for an hour or so and still end up having to make the patient get unnecessary testing done just so their insurance will pay for the test that they *actually* need.

But no doctor has time to sit there and make these phone calls, so they end up having to hire administrative assistants to hang out on the phone and listen to hold music and argue all day. And this then means they have to increase their baseline rates because now they must pay this person purely because insurance companies are ridiculous and stupid (and now they've paid for two tests instead of one).

COVID showed us, as a nation, how controlled doctors are in this country. It showed us that, even though some data was showing that Ivermectin and hydroxychloroquine were likely saving lives and preventing hospitalizations,[2] doctors were not *allowed* to prescribe them because the CDC made them "unapproved" medications to treat that disease. Historically, doctors could use medications for off-label uses whenever they deemed appropriate. But during the pandemic, this was not the case.

It is profoundly troubling how doctors are, quite literally, indoctrinated into the "medical society"—an institution bound by countless unspoken rules. These include never challenging mainstream narratives on hot-button issues like vaccines, dietary guidelines, the use of multiple medications (polypharmacy), the imperative to preserve life at all costs, and adherence to CDC/FDA/WHO/NIH-sanctioned 'truths.'

They are taught throughout school that these large organizations and companies are right—NO MATTER WHAT—and soon become aware of how any doctor that questions the legitimacy of these institutions or their rules is shamed and cancelled.

I talked to several doctors and pharmacists about the effects of remdesivir on our patients, and I had actual medical doctors look at me and tell me that they could see with their own eyes that it was killing people's kidneys and didn't seem to be making a difference against COVID. When I asked why they were still prescribing it, they said that they had to because it was CDC guidelines. When I challenged some of them on this —and why they are just falling in line with this bullshit—they said that they just had to, and that they would get in trouble if they spoke up or didn't follow the guidelines.

This narrative control goes far beyond COVID, though, and has existed for decades. Any doctor who dares step out of line—conducting their own thorough research and reaching conclusions that challenge mainstream healthcare doctrine—risks being denounced, cancelled, and in some cases, terminated with their career destroyed.

Most doctors, unfortunately, just go with the flow and don't have the courage (and support) to make waves.

All of this is to the detriment of the health and wellbeing of everyone.

Healthcare costs have more than tripled since 1970.[3] Why?

Because of the totality of the healthcare industry. All the interconnected elements that make up the healthcare system have gone up in cost, such as technological advances, an aging population, incredibly high drug prices, rising service prices, increased administrative costs (including insurance company profits and CEO salaries), and industry consolidation—each of which contributes to higher overall spending.

It has become impossible for doctors to just do their job. Doctors nowadays are required to not only be experts in healthcare, science, physiology, and clinical diagnostics, but they are also required to be business experts, financial experts, insurance and code experts, lawyers, and counselors all in one! Doctors should get paid way more than they do in most cases (especially primary care docs).

Increasingly, they need to hire support staff so that they can actually get paid by insurance companies so they can make a living. It's a vicious cycle that providers are getting caught in, and many of them are getting the hell out while they can because it's just too much of a pain in the ass to deal with all of this.

The pharmaceutical industry has skyrocketed the cost of patented medications (and smothered the use of generic ones), which in turn has forced insurance companies to increase their premiums and rates. These insurance companies have the real control over your healthcare, and literally dictate what you can and cannot have done for your healthcare needs. Imagine being forced to have a multi-thousand-dollar test that is *clinically unnecessary*, just to be able to get another test that you actually need.

This sounds like insanity to me. And it sounds like insanity to many doctors as well, believe me. They should have the ability to dictate what tests you need or don't need, which medications would best treat your illness, and which treatments will best heal your current problem. Instead, their hands are tied having to appease and deal with health insurance companies and their fuckery.

As doctors leave the profession because of the worsening situation, wait times will become a gigantic problem. I'm not just talking about ER wait times, I'm talking about wait times to get in to see your doctor, surgeon, specialist, or even nurse or nurse practitioner.

Want elective knee replacement surgery so you're not in pain every single day? *Oh, that'll be a two-year wait.*

Want your calluses debrided off your foot so you can walk correctly? *Sure. That'll be 16 weeks out.*

Thinking about following up with a cardiologist after your heart attack? *Word, that'll be nine weeks. But good luck in the meantime. We hope all the interventions we were doing when you were discharged from the hospital are still working well for you.*

Oh, you wanted more pain medication? *That'll be a three-month wait to get in to see your primary care doctor for an assessment, or a six-month wait to get a spot in a pain clinic.*

The average doctor in America finishes school over $200,000 in debt. They also have to pay for malpractice insurance, which varies from $7,000–$40,000 a year depending on their specialty. These are huge costs associated with practicing medicine, and for your average doc just trying to take care of patients in a clinic, the combination of paying for their actual living expenses, school loans, and malpractice insurance doesn't leave much left to buy a yacht with.

The fact that football players make several *million dollars* a year to entertain—but the people who have your actual lives in their hands make less than $250,000 on average—is appalling. I'm not saying all doctors should make millions of dollars a year, but I am saying it should be much more equal than it is.

Doctors are the cornerstone of our healthcare system, but are increasingly burdened by a profession that seems to demand everything and offer little in return. Once revered as healers, they now find themselves trapped in a system that values paperwork over patient care, compliance over clinical judgment, and profit over humanity.

The pressure to appease insurance companies, navigate complex regulations, and practice defensive medicine has stripped many physicians of the joy and purpose that once defined their calling.

Doctors deserve more than our gratitude; they deserve a system that values their expertise, supports their well-being, and allows them to practice medicine as it was meant to be practiced—with integrity, compassion, curiosity, and care. It's time to stop treating physicians as cogs in a machine and start treating them as the irreplaceable professionals they are.

The world needs doctors.

Actually, the world needs *good, happy, and fulfilled* doctors.

CHAPTER 8

PARTNERING FOR PROGRESS
HEALTHCARE ADMINISTRATION AND THE FRONTLINES

HEALTHCARE ADMINISTRATION IS a complex and sensitive subject, particularly for those of us who work on the frontlines.

As healthcare providers, we often feel unseen and unheard by the leadership in C-suites or upper management. From our perspective, people sit in their offices and have meetings about what we do but have no actual *concept* of what we do. Many of these decision-makers are far removed from the realities of patient care, and that disconnect can be a problem. For one, policies and procedures are created without a full understanding of how they will work in the real world, and while they may look great on paper, they often lead to frustration, inefficiency, and even delays in patient care.

This disconnect isn't malicious, but it can sometimes feel that way. Administrators are tasked with managing budgets, maintaining compliance with regulatory requirements, and ensuring the financial stability of their institutions. These are huge responsibilities.

But the challenge is this: how can leaders make decisions

that affect frontline staff and patients without truly understanding the work being done?

Leaders at all levels—whether middle management or C-suite executives—need to step out of their offices and spend more time with the people who are the backbone of their organizations. Immersing themselves in the day-to-day realities of their staff would provide valuable insights into the challenges and successes of their facilities.

Imagine if a hospital CEO spent a week shadowing their employees: following a nurse through a twelve-hour shift; observing a CNA (certified nursing assistant) as they tend to patients' basic needs; or assisting a physical therapist during a rehab session. Picture them following a doctor, living the reality of having to make split-second decisions that can alter the course of a human life.

They might witness an ER team managing multiple critical cases simultaneously, or see the emotional toll an ICU nurse endures as they hold the hand of a dying patient.

These experiences would undoubtedly lead to better-informed decisions by leadership with profound consequences for the well-being of both staff and patients.

It's easy to sit at a long wooden table with water glasses and note pads and say something like:

> "Well, the acuity of patients in the ICUs has dropped since COVID. So, our nurses should be able to handle at least three patients each, and do not need CNAs to help them anymore. Therefore, we've decided we will have one CNA who works as the unit secretary and CNA for day shift, and none during night shift. This isn't a big deal on their workload and should save us approximately 6 bajillion dollars. Let the unit directors know

that they have to tell their CNAs they don't have jobs as of tonight at 7 pm, those that show up for work will be sent home."

I use this as an example because it literally (well, with some paraphrasing) happened in my hospital.

One day in 2022, we were told we were no longer having full-time CNA coverage, and that they don't need to come back to work tomorrow and will be reached out to by management for possible options to get some more hours.

This is a decision that could only be made by people who do not take care of patients. While most days have some periods of downtime in the ICU; when it's busy, it is DANGEROUS if nurses are overworked and trying to do the job of both a nurse and a CNA.

Business and management knowledge and expertise is essential to lead effectively in healthcare. But it's not enough. Administrators also need a foundational understanding of the patient care experience.

One way to bridge this gap is to prioritize hiring administrators with hands-on clinical experience. This would bring a level of insight that cannot be taught in a classroom or gleaned from financial reports. Whether they are former nurses, doctors, therapists, or CNAs—they will understand the realities of patient care because they've *lived it*. They know the physical and emotional demands of the work, the challenges of triaging your daily tasks, and the importance of teamwork.

This doesn't discount the value of business expertise—managing budgets, navigating regulations, and optimizing operations. But the best leaders are those who can combine their business-sense with a deep understanding of the human side of healthcare. They recognize that their role is not just to oversee operations and figures, but to support the people who make those operations possible.

By ensuring that leadership roles are filled by people with both clinical and administrative expertise, we can create a healthcare system that is more empathetic, efficient, and effective. Leaders who have walked in the shoes of their staff are better equipped to craft policies that are both practical and impactful.

Some aspects of healthcare are the most regulated sectors in the world, and for good reason. Patient safety and quality of care depend on strict standards. However, not all policies are created equal. Some are based on outdated theories, while others are overly burdensome and not realistic for actual patient care. State and federal regulations play a huge role in shaping hospital policies, and compliance with their regulations is non-negotiable.

Compliance with CMS (Centers for Medicare and Medicaid) regulations is assessed by state surveyors, who are often experienced healthcare professionals. They meticulously review patient charts and facility practices to ensure that standards are met. These surveys are completed on a set schedule—typically every three years—to ensure your facility is complying with their regulations. While these surveys are essential for maintaining accountability, they also highlight an important issue: the gap between regulatory requirements and real-world application.

As someone who has served as an administrator, I understand the pressure that comes with these state surveys. Every detail has to be perfect; every chart meticulously documented; and every intervention flawlessly executed. They go through charts with a fine-toothed comb and make sure each of these patients received the level of care required to qualify for reimbursement, and that everything was documented appropriately.

One oversight can result in citations, financial penalties, or even the loss of Medicare and Medicaid funding. If your facility did anything that caused a patient harm, you are held liable and will have financial consequences.

While I understand the need to hold facilities accountable, complications occur, side effects happen, and unwanted outcomes are unavoidable. Sometimes a healthcare provider may have been too frazzled, too busy, or too overwhelmed and didn't document a certain case perfectly. Maybe—if the system wasn't based on penalizing hospitals financially—they wouldn't have to be so focused on the bottom line all the time.

I've seen first-hand the powerful effect of leadership style on the ethos of a hospital.

One CEO I worked under made it a point to know all employees by name, walk the halls regularly, and ask how he could help. He was approachable, engaged, and genuinely invested in the well-being of his staff. His leadership style created a positive, motivated workplace where employees felt valued and supported.

On the other hand, I've also worked under leaders who remained distant and detached. They only appeared during meetings or when a crisis happened. Their lack of visibility and engagement created an environment of distrust and disconnection, leaving staff feeling undervalued and unsupported.

True leadership is about more than making decisions from behind a desk. It's about building relationships, understanding the challenges your team faces, and empowering them to succeed. Administrators should prioritize addressing systemic issues such as staffing shortages, burnout, and inadequate pay. These are not just important concerns, fixing them is essential for retaining talented professionals and ensuring the sustainability of our healthcare system.

Administrators and staff must work as a cohesive team,

recognizing that every role is essential—from the housekeeper to the CEO. Boards of directors are notoriously filled with retired, inactive people and executives. A typical one might consist of that doc who retired 15 years ago, the retired director of nurses from ten years ago, a layperson off the streets (this is a legal requirement), the CEO of course, and probably a PRN occupational therapist who works one day every two weeks on the hospital's rehab floor.

These folks have little to absolutely no understanding of the *current* inner workings of areas such as critical care, the operating room, or the emergency room.

I think a possible solution is to ensure that at least half of the members of every healthcare facility's board of directors are current, active, full-time employees. I realize there is a reason for outsiders to be involved too, but at least half should be people who have real, insider information on the functioning of the entity itself. These frontline voices can provide invaluable insights, helping to create policies that are practical, effective, and grounded in reality.

One of the most glaring inequities in healthcare today is the wage disparity between administrators and frontline workers. CEOs and other high-level administrators often earn six-figure, and sometimes even seven-figure, salaries annually. This applies to not just hospitals, but to insurance companies, pharmaceutical companies, and equipment manufacturers.

In contrast, many healthcare workers—those who perform the physically and emotionally grueling work of direct patient care—struggle to make ends meet on hourly wages that do not reflect the intensity of their responsibilities.

This wage gap sends a stark message, whether intentional or not: the work of those on the frontlines is less important. It is undervalued. This creates an environment where staff feel expendable, while those in administrative positions, often far removed from the day-to-day realities of their own business, are paid much more. The effects of this disparity go beyond morale. Underpaid workers are more likely to experience burnout, financial stress, and create turnover, all of which directly impact patient care.

When nurses, CNAs, and other critical staff are overworked and undercompensated, it becomes nearly impossible to deliver the level of care patients deserve.

This gap also highlights a systemic imbalance in how we define value in healthcare. While administrators play a necessary role in keeping hospitals running smoothly, the lifeblood of any healthcare organization is its frontline workers. They are the ones who interact with patients, manage emergencies, and provide comfort during life's most vulnerable moments. Without them, no amount of administrative genius could keep a hospital functional.

To bridge this divide, healthcare organizations must take a hard look at their compensation structures. CEOs and other executives deserve to be compensated for their expertise and responsibilities, but not at the expense of those who make patient care possible.

One solution could be implementing wage caps or linking executive compensation to metrics that include employee satisfaction, retention rates, and patient outcomes—not just financial performance or customer satisfaction rates.

Additionally, healthcare organizations should prioritize raising wages for frontline staff, ensuring they are paid fairly for the vital work they do. The point is, we should have a healthcare system where compensation reflects the essential contributions of every employee, from the CNA who provides hands-on care to the CEO who oversees operations.

Ultimately, the goal is to create a healthcare system where

everyone—administrators, staff, and patients—feels valued and supported.

To the administrators who hold the reins of healthcare institutions: you have the power to create profound change. Your decisions ripple through every corner of your organization, shaping the experiences of both patients and staff. Doing something as small as denying your own bonus so that your employees can get a better raise or a bonus themselves would make an enormous difference in people's lives.

The frontline workers who pour their hearts into this profession deserve to feel supported, respected, and understood. They are not just numbers on a spreadsheet or statistics in a report; they are the backbone of healthcare, the ones who ensure that your mission is fulfilled every single day. By stepping into their world, by listening to their struggles and celebrating their triumphs, you can bridge the gap that so often divides us. You can lead not just from the boardroom but from the heart, creating a culture where every employee feels seen, heard, and valued.

Together, we can create a healthcare system that not only heals patients but uplifts everyone within it—a system built on empathy, collaboration, and a shared commitment to excellence.

CHAPTER 9
PREDATORY POWER
HOW BIG PHARMA HOLDS OUR HEALTH HOSTAGE

PHARMACEUTICAL COMPANIES HAVE BECOME TOO big for their britches. Along with Big Tech (Apple, Google, etc.), Big Finance, and Big Oil companies, Big Pharma is undoubtedly one of the most powerful entities in the world.

The power that they wield over most people's daily lives is truly astounding. These companies can influence international drug prices, access to medications, and global health initiatives. They hold monopolies over intellectual property that controls the production and sale of life-saving medications. They are able to shape the healthcare system and national policy decisions by spending billions of dollars lobbying the federal government. This allows them to sway and influence drug prices, patents for drugs, and overall access to healthcare.

We as Americans have been gaslit and manipulated by Big Pharma and it has come at the cost of our health as a nation.

Big Pharma has been accused of putting profits over health for decades. One glaringly problematic practice is the tendency to spend significantly more money on sales and marketing than they do into the actual research and development of the drug itself. America's Health Insurance Plans (AHIP) is a trade association whose mission it is to advocate for a more equitable, affordable, and sustainable healthcare system. They estimate that Big Pharma spends approximately 37% more on direct-to-consumer advertising than they do on the research and development of their medications.[1]

This shows that they are more concerned with the amount of drugs sold than they are with developing new formulations to treat or cure diseases.

In the past, drugs were mostly only marketed to doctors. Drug reps would go from town to town and visit doctors' offices or homes and sell their products directly to them. This kept a lot of power in the hands and judgement of doctors, which was a good thing. Doctors were the only ones who had the capability of selecting, out of their available supplies in their office, the appropriate drug for their patient. And if they didn't have what they needed, they either had to send a carrier to a major city or figure something else out.

In 1997, the FDA changed their guidelines to allow direct-to-consumer advertising by drug companies. There had been some regulations since the 1980s regarding marketing for prescriptions, but until 1997 the regulations had been very restrictive, making advertising difficult for drug companies.[2] The only countries to this day that allow this are the US and New Zealand.

Lauren McGrath of Princeton University notes that this "deregulation" didn't empower consumers to make informed choices; it empowered pharmaceutical companies to weaponize marketing.[3]

Enter Purdue Pharma.

In 1996, they introduced OxyContin—the first narcotic medication marketed directly to consumers—and changed the game forever. Purdue convinced the public that pain, of any kind, deserved treatment with their drug, reframing pain as the "fifth vital sign." Their aggressive campaigns hammered home the idea that chronic pain—which could often be managed with nonpharmaceutical interventions or over-the-counter meds—required OxyContin, a potent opioid. They even claimed it was non-addictive, often stating that addiction was "very rare."[4]

Spoiler alert: look around, it wasn't.

Purdue hammered home the idea that getting treated for chronic aches and pains—that could almost always be treated with nonpharmaceutical interventions or even Tylenol or Advil—really needed to be treated with this "top-tier" painkiller. They particularly promoted it as the most effective drug out there for managing chronic pain issues. As we have witnessed, the demand for the drug was unprecedented.

Imagine being a 75-year-old veteran suffering from chronic pain. A magic pill promising relief? Of course you'd want it.

Purdue didn't stop at advertising; they incentivized doctors with coupons for free prescriptions and funded thousands of educational sessions promoting narcotics for chronic pain. The result? An opioid epidemic that has claimed countless lives. People were instantly hooked on not only the actual pills, but the idea of the pills themselves. Purdue's actions seemed to be deliberate, calculated, and devastating. They and companies like them likely bear significant responsibility for the crisis we're still suffering.

Fast-forward to today, and Big Pharma's marketing tactics have only become even more predatory. Turn on the TV, and you'll see ads featuring happy couples in infinity pools, selling the illusion that a pill is the key to a better life. This constant barrage has shifted the power dynamic in healthcare. Patients now walk into doctor's offices expecting—*no, demanding*—prescriptions. Granted, medications have been the backbone of medicine forever. But not in the same way.

Usually, if the doctor believed a medication would help you, they would prescribe one. If they thought something more like a splint, a change in diet, or bed rest for a time would work, they would prescribe that. Doctors have years and years of rigorous medical education to prepare them for taking care of people. A lay person's knowledge about medications and their uses for treating diseases does not compare to that of a doctor. Big pharma has been trying to convince uneducated, lay people that they know just as much as doctors do for about 30 years now, and it has created many problems, side effects, and deaths.

Which is exactly what Big Pharma wants.

Pharmaceutical companies didn't just stumble into this power—they bought it. Lobbyists from companies like Pfizer and Merck poured millions into convincing Congress that direct-to-consumer advertising would empower patients and increase awareness about health issues. They claimed this would give people more control over their own lives and health. Eventually, their money and slogans got through to Congress and have led us to the rotten system we have now.[5] A system where manipulation masquerades as empowerment.

I believe we should look to other countries when it comes to the direct-to-consumer advertising of drugs. Most have banned direct-to-consumer advertising, recognizing the harm it would cause and have not allowed drug company money to corrupt safety policy.

In the US, the direct marketing of prescription drugs to the public has led to almost unlimited budgets used by these companies to exploit and mislead the general public. It has also led to astronomically high prices for drugs that cost pennies to produce. It is impossible to know how many people have been killed or permanently harmed by these drugs, and that is frightening.

But in America, Big Pharma's dollars speak louder than public health concerns.

Then there's the issue of drug pricing. Americans (and our health insurance companies) pay higher prices for medications than anywhere else in the world. According to hhs.gov, Americans spent a staggering $603 billion on medications in 2021.[6] Pharma companies use many different strategies to continue to keep drug prices high and nonnegotiable. One of the most egregious ways they do this is by influencing patent protections, which allow them to maintain monopolies over their drugs for many many years.

Patents usually last 20 years, but this includes the development and research years. To keep extending patents, most pharma companies will "evergreen" their product. By making very slight, pointless changes to the chemical structure of the drug, they can apply for a new patent. This allows them to continue their monopoly over the medication and to charge whatever inflated price they want.[7]

Evergreening is also used by Big Pharma to prevent generic drugs from being developed. This prevents any competition in the drug marketplace and allows these companies to continue to take advantage of high drug prices.

A key case of this that is not well known by the public is AstraZeneca's Prilosec and Nexium.[8] These two drugs are considered "blockbuster" drugs, drugs that created $1 billion or more in revenue a year for the manufacturer. They are both frequently prescribed proton pump inhibitors (PPIs) used to reduce stomach acid and treat conditions like stomach ulcers and reflux.

AstraZeneca knew that its hit drug Prilosec was going to lose its patent protection in 2001. They decided to evergreen it: they tweaked a tiny chemical component and marketed it as a completely new and improved medication: Nexium. Their advertisements for it claimed that it was more effective and had fewer side effects than Prilosec. In fact, most studies showed that it was almost exactly the same in terms of effectiveness and reported that it had *more* side effects than its sister drug.[9]

AstraZeneca heavily promoted Nexium to both doctors and consumers and encouraged everyone taking Prilosec to transition over to their "new and improved" medication before the patent for Prilosec expired. This allowed AstraZeneca to continue to charge an inflated price for their "new" drug Nexium, which was chemically almost identical to the generic forms of Prilosec that were now available.

Like its precursor, Nexium also became a blockbuster drug and made the company billions of more dollars.

What a great scam . . .

Attempts to rein in these practices, such as limiting formulary exclusions, have largely backfired. These policies aim to limit the number of medications that insurance companies can deny payment for. There are several states that have placed restrictions on certain classes of medications, such as cancer drugs, mental health drugs, and autoimmune disease treatments. Their goal is to ensure that every patient has access to any medication within those classes, regardless of cost.

While the intention is noble the reality is these policies often lead to higher premiums and out-of-pocket costs. Why? Because pharmaceutical companies manipulate the system to stay on formularies, driving up prices. If we can stop these companies from monopolizing medications for decade upon decade, we would very likely see an overall decrease in medication prices over time.

The real solution lies in addressing patent manipulation and breaking up monopolies, but Big Pharma's lobbying efforts make that a herculean task.

Another fundamental issue with Big Pharma is their fraudulent activity within the research and clinical trials sector. Time and again, pharmaceutical companies have been caught withholding data, skewing results, and outright lying to the public. There have been many high-profile cases over the years where pharma companies have had to shell out billions of dollars for misleading the public or purposely withholding data showing poor outcomes of their drugs.

In 2005, The *New England Journal of Medicine* published several articles accusing pharma giant Merck of withholding data about the drug Vioxx (an NSAID pain reliever).[10] There were several studies on Vioxx that indicated it significantly increased the risks of heart attack and stroke. To hide this, Merck only published studies showing the drug in a positive light and suppressed those telling the truth—that the drug was dangerous.

It is estimated that Vioxx caused 88,000 heart attacks and at least 38,000 deaths in its few years on the market.[11] Merck was eventually required to pay out almost $5 billion to settle legal claims.[12]

This is just one example of unethical behavior that has caused large-scale death and suffering of innocent people. More recently, there have been similar lawsuits against another Big Pharma giant, Gilead, regarding the medication Remdesivir.[13]

As I mentioned in Chapter 1, several studies—including one conducted by the WHO—have found that Remdesivir does not reduce mortality in COVID-19 patients.[14] These studies, combined with others that indicate that Remdesivir increases the risk of kidney failure, have prompted several lawsuits against Gilead.

For the same reasons, the WHO issued a recommendation *against* the use of Remdesivir in COVID-19 patients in 2020. But the US decided to go against this and made it the drug of choice to treat COVID-19, despite its serious side effects and lack of efficacy in decreasing deaths. They claimed they did this because a study in the *New England Journal of Medicine* showed that, in some cases, Remdesivir could decrease patient hospital stays from 15 to ten days.[15]

I understand the desire to decrease hospitalization time, especially during a pandemic with hospitals at capacity across the nation. But if we are having multiple conflicting results on a medication's effectiveness and safety, I don't believe it should be the drug of choice during a global pandemic.

(A side note: It is important to note that the studies relied upon by the CDC and NIH were *funded by the NIH*. Make of that what you will.)

Further legal issues are plaguing Gilead because of the cost of Remdesivir. The price point *per dose* of Remdesivir is $520 for private insurance and $390 for US government insurances such as Medicare. So, for a five-day course, that is $3,120 and $2,340 respectively. These numbers are from Gilead's own press release about the cost of their new drug.[16] It is reported by the company itself that Remdesivir has made them over $16 billion since 2020.

How is a drug that was developed to save lives during a global pandemic—and largely funded by our own tax dollars—so unbelievably expensive? This is yet another example of Big Pharma's predatory, unethical, and shameful behavior.

There are many more unethical actions by Big Pharma that could—and should—be explored, but the final issue I want to address here is their manipulation of public policy. They do this by having *very* powerful lobbyists with *very* deep pockets.

According to Duke University, lobbying is the ability of a company, individual, or entity to petition the government to act in their benefit.[17] Generally—except maybe for the inclusion of "company"—this is a positive thing that allows people to participate in and influence governmental decisions, policies, and regulations to benefit the public.

But this is not the case with Big Pharma.

Big Pharma uses lobbying and political contributions to sway governmental decisions solely to benefit their own pockets. As the top lobbying spender of any industry, they have spent over $5.83 billion from 1998 to 2023 influencing our government's policy towards health and medications.[18]

One of the most important areas they have kept under their control is the ability of the Federal Government to be able to negotiate drug prices. Under current law, Medicare is not allowed to negotiate drug prices—they simply have to pay whatever price the pharmaceutical companies charge them.

Pharma companies have also lobbied hard against putting price caps on any class of medications, arguing that it will decrease the incentive to develop new drugs. While this could be true to some extent, lobbies like this are one of the sole reasons why healthcare is so damned expensive in this country—more than double the average of other high-income nations.[19]

Another big area of lobbying is that of patent protection. On top of evergreening, as discussed above, Big Pharma companies lobby the US Patent and Trademark Office to grant them overly broad patents so they can keep their patents (aka monopolies) for longer. These effectively block any competition and allow them to keep prices consistently high. There have been several articles published regarding this issue in popular sources such as the *Harvard Business Review*.[20]

The FDA is a government agency that is supposed to keep us safe from harm potentially caused by these pharmaceutical companies. But there is a huge conflict of interest: a large portion of the funding for the FDA—about 45% ($2.7 billion in "industry user fees" in 2020)—comes directly from Big Pharma itself.[21]

The *New York Times* has published an article about the conflicts of interest this can pose.[22] Many critics of the FDA argue that it allows drugs to be approved way too quickly, and without the proper proof of safety, because they fear losing these "industry user fees." I find it utterly revolting that this happens right under our noses, and no one ever does anything about it. The FDA should be purely government funded because it is *clearly* a conflict of interest to have funding by the very companies it is meant to regulate. Self-regulation in a profit-driven industry is a joke.

I am disgusted by many other things surrounding these pharmaceutical companies. Their deep pockets just continue to get deeper at the expense of our health, and it just shouldn't be this way. I don't like complaining about things without offering potential solutions, but this is a complex problem. While I support the need for an incentive (i.e., profit) for scientists to perform ground-breaking research into potentially life-saving medications, I don't want these medications to cost more than a HOUSE for patients in need.

I believe that if you need a medication, you should have unfettered access to it, no matter what. Drugs should be developed for public health, not profit.

One solution to consider is interventions to stop people needing these medications in the first place. Obviously, in many cases—such as people who have received an organ transplant and need immunosuppressants so they don't die—these medications are an absolute necessity. But the vast majority of people on chronic medications (such as reflux meds, cholesterol meds, or blood pressure meds)—and there are tens of millions of people on such drugs—probably wouldn't need them long-term if they made different lifestyle choices.

Although many people make an effort to be healthy, a major problem is that they lack understanding of what "healthy" actually means. Being healthy is not just the lack of being obese. It is ensuring that you are feeding your body with real, whole foods and are exercising appropriately.

Being healthy is *changing your entire lifestyle* to preserve your health and not die.

Dr. Michael Greger has a series of phenomenal books dedicated to healing your body with food and exercise, rather than pills and medical interventions. These include *How Not to Diet, How Not to Die,* and *How Not to Age.*[23] This man is a real doctor that has dedicated his life to educating the public on the fact that what we put into our mouths is the most important decision we will ever make. He has watched his family members go from being on several prescription drugs with life-limiting diagnoses (like end-stage heart disease), to living twenty five more healthy years, on little to no medications, just by changing their diet and lifestyle.

If we, as a nation, embraced such a mindset, we could dismantle Big Pharma's grip on our lives. By choosing whole, unprocessed foods and prioritizing wellness, we could reverse countless chronic diseases, extend our life expectancy, and reclaim our collective power. Yes, changing our habits—and challenging the processed food industry—may feel daunting, but it's far more achievable than we've been led to believe.

Big Pharma has placed profit over people for far too long. It's time for us to take back control, make sustainable changes, and prioritize our health above all else— especially the profits of mega-corporations.

CHAPTER 10

A SYSTEM THAT PRETENDS TO CARE

HOW INSURANCE FAILS THE SICK AND REWARDS THE POWERFUL

THE AMERICAN HEALTH insurance business had honest and humble beginnings.

Insurance and tech expert Ellen Lichtenstein wrote an in-depth article on the history of health insurance that provides some very helpful insight on how we got to the system we have now.[1]

Essentially, in the early 1900s, welfare and government programs were rare, so some banks and private companies kept "sickness funds." These were stockpiles of money set aside by banks or private companies to pay their members or employees an amount of money to replace their lost income if they became sick or injured.

Workers' compensation programs evolved from earlier sickness fund systems, enabling employers to provide proper reimbursement to employees injured on the job. Companies purchased insurance plans—often through state programs—which allowed them to support their employees in times of need. Neither of these programs was mandatory; some companies back then wanted their employees to live healthy lives and be able to earn a living. It was much more feasible at the time because these programs were affordable and worthwhile for companies, helping them retain their employees and build loyalty.

During the Great Depression of the 1930s, hospitals faced severe financial challenges. In response, they devised an innovative solution: signing up patients or their employers as "members" and charging a monthly fee—essentially a premium—in exchange for guaranteed coverage of certain hospital services. As you might expect, incoming payments exceeded treatment costs, so the hospitals started to see some extra income.

These programs were soon deemed health insurance programs akin to life insurance, and this is when our modern insurance industry blossomed into the dumpster fire it is today.

During World War II, the government passed legislation stating that the value of employer-provided health insurance would not be counted as part of an employee's taxable wages, but instead treated as a separate, non-taxable benefit. At this time, employers were offering health insurance voluntarily as a genuine benefit to attract and retain workers—it was not required by law or mandated by the government.

Insurance benefit programs soon separated from the hospitals to become new companies, and modern insurance companies were born. Initially, all these companies offered their benefits at the same premium prices, regardless of your health risk or preexisting conditions. That's because it was a *benefit*.

However, soon after their conception as the companies they are today, they began offering healthier people better premiums and charging sicker, and higher-risk people, more—like most life insurance companies still do today. For this reason, the elderly who were past their working years and likely made less money than they had (or none at all) were stuck with the highest premium rates.

Medicare was founded to protect the elderly from the price-gouging of the private health insurance companies by automatically providing them with healthcare coverage once they reached a certain age and had paid into the system through a tax on their wages. Similarly, Medicaid was also born at this time and was designed to protect those who were disabled or very poor.

According to the US Department of Health and Human Services website, the difference was (and still is) that Medicaid was not mandated into every state; it was the state's choice to either participate, not participate, or partially participate in the Medicaid benefit program.[2] If you are on Medicaid, you generally have very little to no out-of-pocket expense for any healthcare needs.

By the 1980s, there were different types of more complex insurance plans, such as Health Maintenance Organizations (HMOs), Preferred Provider Organizations (PPOs), and Point of Service (POS) plans.* By this point, there were already many problems in our health insurance world, including the high number of uninsured, rising healthcare prices with rising premium costs, and accessibility to healthcare for the poor or destitute.

I found these shocking statistics on kff.org—an "independent source for health policy research, polling, and journalism": In 2010, 46.5 million Americans were uninsured because the cost of premiums had risen to unprecedented levels.[3] In 2022, thanks mostly to the Affordable Care Act (ACA), the unin-

---

* Health Maintenance Organization (HMO): Requires members to use a network of providers and get referrals for specialists. Preferred Provider Organization (PPO): Offers more flexibility to see any provider, with lower costs for using in-network providers. Point of Service (POS): Combines HMO and PPO features; requires a primary care doctor and referrals, but allows some out-of-network care.

sured portion of the population was massively reduced to 25.6 million. Most uninsured Americans (64%) say that the high cost of coverage is the main reason they do not have health insurance. Most are in very low-income, working-class families, are generally people of color, and may not be citizens.

Although we now have fewer people with no health insurance, the accessibility of healthcare in America is extremely one-sided. If you walk into a hospital or doctor's office with private insurance, you are frequently treated *better* than you are with Medicare or Medicaid. The reimbursement levels are higher with private insurance (like we discussed in the last chapter on Big Pharma), and therefore there is an unconscious (or conscious) bias toward these patients.

I have witnessed this many times in my career. A typical response might be, "Well, they have United insurance, so we should be able to get them placed in a really nice facility," which has been said to me more times than I can count. I have seen patients have prolonged hospital stays because a bed they were promised by a facility was given to someone else with better insurance reimbursement rates. I have physically been in facilities that take primarily Medicare/Medicaid patients and facilities that take primarily private insurances, and I will tell you there is a *major difference* in the quality of care and quality of the physical building.

Our current broken system has caused this disparity, and it is shameful.

So, why do we even need health insurance? Like, how come it's not possible for us to just go to the doctor when we are sick, pay a standard fee, and get the treatments that we need for a normal price? Why is it that we have allowed the costs in our medical system to rise so astronomically without holding companies accountable? I address these questions in Chapter 12.

Hospitals have notoriously overcharged patients. If you ask for an itemized bill from your hospital stay, your eyes will bug right out of your head. I've seen so many posts from people online that show the line-item breakdown of the charges from their hospital stay, and it is just shocking. I have also witnessed a disturbing number of times where a bill mysteriously shrinks once the patient asks to see exactly what they're charged for.

For example, I saw a post on Facebook by a woman in New York who had just given birth, and she was charged $40 to hold her own newborn baby. Another charged a patient $600 to remove stitches. (Removing stitches usually takes less than five minutes.) Or how about this one: being charged $1,000 an hour for observation. I mean, I understand that hospitals have huge overhead costs, but *a thousand dollars an hour?*

And how has this happened? Where did we go wrong?

I'll tell you where: No one has held companies accountable.

In America—with its capitalist foundation and socialized elements—companies have the right to come up with services, technologies, and other products, and sell them on the free market for whatever they deem it to be worth, right?

So, if I am a scientist and come up with a new technology that can save lives, I have the right to charge essentially what I want for it, since it improves outcomes, and the industry will want access to my idea. The problem with this is that it gives the creators (or the people with the patents), the ability to charge WAY more for the product than it costs to make, with no accountability and no regulations. We've already discussed this in terms of drug patents and Big Pharma in the previous chapter.

Now, are there regulations on all the other steps involved in developing medical equipment, techniques, supplies, or medications?

Absolutely. Which means the government is choosing to

step in where they want to, but not at all when it comes to cost. They are basically saying that we must follow all of their rules and regulations for producing these items and using them on humans, but that any dollar amount can be charged for them.

I have a weird feeling this might have something to do with lobbyists and large kickbacks to government agencies for keeping the pricing basically regulation-free . . . ?

Hospitals and distribution companies state that their prices are "industry standard" and include middlemen that need to get paid as well. I understand that there are several hands that touch these medical devices before they end up in the patient's room, but dang! A bag of saline costs about $1 to produce, but by the time it's charged to the patient, the price ranges from $100–$500 a bag.[4] A *New York Times* investigation in 2013 found that hospitals were charging markups of 100 to 200 times the manufacturer's price.

The reality is that behind the scenes, deals are struck, hospitals and other facilities receive discounts, and mutual favors are exchanged—all while these companies continue to make money hand over fist. Hospitals and healthcare facilities are constantly dealing with mergers and acquisitions and attempts to save costs to increase profits by any means necessary. These deals made probably go something like this:

> IV fluid company: Hey, distribution company, do you need IV fluid for the hospitals you service? Cool. We are charging you $4 a bag for saline to cover our production costs and wages for employees at wholesale cost.

> Distribution company: Thanks! We will charge the hospital $20 for this bag of saline because we have to cover gas for our trucks, maintenance, and the truck drivers' wages.

> Hospital: Okay, we will then charge the patient and their insurance company $447 for that bag of saline because we have to pay the distribution staff within our hospital to bring the saline up to the floors, also the nurse's/doctor's salary to give the medication and monitor them, also the electricity for the hospital, also the mortgage for the hospital, and also . . . ummm . . . because we can.

Whatever the overheads they have to include, if it honestly costs them $447 to obtain and give a bag of saline, we are so screwed. I have no solutions if that's the case. But I have a strong suspicion that they are increasing the prices *just a little bit* to make some money. A lot of money. I understand they are businesses and need to make money, but this markup seems a tad over the top, wouldn't you say?

And let's not forget that insurance companies are *allowing* this incredible markup of such a simple product. Insurance companies negotiate with hospitals for these things, so the hospital's reimbursement can change according to their deductibles, insurance plans, and copayments. It's incredibly complex and difficult to track and understand. Which makes it much easier to get away with.

Insurance companies do technically have industry standards that they follow when it comes to what they will cover for each item during a hospitalization or any healthcare encounter. These are usually set by what Medicare or Medicaid will typically pay and include those regulated formulary exclusions I spoke about earlier, where they cannot deny certain types of treatments and medications.

That's fine, but what they don't really make clear is that they will cover a *portion* of these treatments and medications and then leave the patient responsible for the rest.

When my youngest son was around 14 months old, he

became seriously ill. What started as a mild cold escalated over the course of a month into something much more concerning. I tried everything I could at home to avoid taking him to the emergency room—I'm a nurse, after all, and I felt confident in my ability to manage his care. But one night, his breathing became so labored that I couldn't get his oxygen levels above the low 80s. I knew then that we had crossed a line.

I took him to our local community hospital, and we were seen in the emergency room. We were there for about an hour. After about 30 minutes in the waiting room, they brought him back, flushed his nose with saline, suctioned the mucus, waited a few minutes, saw that his oxygen had improved to the 90s, and discharged us.

A week later, he deteriorated further. At one point, I was laying in the middle of the living room floor with him at 4 am. I had basically not slept for almost three weeks at this point because I was terrified that he would stop breathing. So, I would lay with him on the hard floor, where his lungs worked the best. I was staring at his tiny chest working so hard for each breath and obsessively checking his oxygen levels.

He was lethargic, he was gray, and he was laying there moaning. By 5 am, it had been about three hours that his oxygen hadn't risen above 80%, despite all my efforts of suctioning, percussion, medications, sitting in the bathroom with the shower steaming him, increasing his oxygen level, and holding his whimpering body. I decided that we were driving to Denver to go to Children's Hospital, where they could help save my baby because I was at my wit's end.

The drive was over two hours, and I was terrified the whole way. Once there, he was admitted with bilateral pneumonia, influenza, bilateral ear infections, and sepsis. His tiny body had simply run out of energy to keep fighting. After two nights in the hospital, with oxygen support, IV antibiotics, and deep suctioning, he began to get better and eventually made a full recovery.

About two months later, I received two bills. The total from Children's Hospital for the ER, hospital stay, and treatments was about $2,500. I was shocked at how reasonable that seemed. Then I opened the bill from the local ER.

For that single, one-hour visit, we were charged $8,700.

I called my insurance company, expecting some kind of mistake. But the representative explained that I had a $7,000 deductible, and that this bill, outrageous as it was, had been processed correctly.

"Honestly, it's not that bad," she said. I wasn't upset about my deductible. I had accepted that as part of my plan. What I could not accept was being charged nearly $9,000 for a single hour in the ER, during which the only intervention was suctioning with ten milliliters of saline.

When I requested an itemized bill, I received what is shown in Table 1.

No one should have to pay nearly nine thousand dollars for what was essentially a nasal suction. And yet, because he was coded as a "Level 2" emergency visit—a designation that implies significant risk, my family was held responsible for the vast majority of the cost.

Description	Charge
ER visit Level 2: respiratory distress, pediatric	$8,000
ER respiratory interventions, pediatric	$1,400
ER physician consultation, pediatric	$500
ER administrative fees	$350
Total visit	$10,250
Insurance payment	$1,550
Patient responsibility	$8,700

Table 1 My itemized bill from my local ER.

I knew as a nurse that this level of coding was inaccurate. I fought it. I made phone calls to both the hospital and the insurance company, explaining exactly what was done during our visit. But the hospital refused to change the level of care coding, citing the triage nurse's initial designation.

And so we were stuck.

By the way, this was when I had insurance through the ACA (Affordable Care Act) portal. My premium at the time was around $680 a month for my family of four, and that was the cheapest plan with one of the higher deductibles of $7,000. So, I was paying $8,160 a year in premiums, plus was responsible for a $7,000 deductible, PLUS whatever else was denied by the insurance company. My other option was a $5,000 deductible for $900 a month, or a $3,000 deductible for $1,200 a month.

There was no way I could afford those premium rates, so I went with the lowest one. Oh, also, if you didn't know, all these rates through the ACA are based on your income, so they base your premium rates on how much money you make. Because I am a RN, I am categorized as a "middle class" earner and my premiums were on the higher side.

This personal experience with the healthcare system on the patient side really opened my eyes. We have to watch our backs, be on our toes, and fight for our right to have affordable healthcare in one of the richest countries in the world. It seems very backward to me.

As an outsider, you would think that the American government really has its people's health as a priority. I mean, they have the Food and Drug Administration, Office of Disease Prevention and Health Promotion, and Centers for Disease Control and Prevention. Then there is the World Health Organization that they are very active in.

But let's be real here; what do these agencies actually do for us as the average American?

Well, given their flip-flopping on policies, mandates, and

requirements during the pandemic, the CDC has proven to be pretty unreliable and crazy.

If you go to their website, they have a 'National Health Initiatives, Strategies & Action Plans' section. This lovely ball of "education" has several links to planning documents that "address the nation's most pressing health problems." These documents are not user friendly and are certainly not accessible to or understandable by the average American.

We all know that the number-one killer of Americans is heart disease, right? Like, hundreds of thousands of people a year die from cardiac issues, mostly from lifestyle and dietary choices. Well, the CDC has started many programs to fight heart disease over recent decades, and there is a link to these strategies for improvement on the heart disease section of their website . . . except I noted that it wasn't updated for almost a decade until May 2024.

In 2020, after a decline in deaths due to heart disease of 9% between 2010–2019, the rate increased by 4%.[6] This means that approximately five years of improvement was essentially erased by the pandemic and all of its bullshit.

The FDA does its best to regulate food and drug labels, but companies find ways around this all the time. They are also pretty busy with regulating the pharmaceutical industry for humans and animals, food production and the food chain, the cosmetology industry, and anything that emits radiation. That is A LOT of things to be the number one authority on in the nation.

It's fascinating to me the amount of power the government has over certain things, but when it comes to others—like the price of healthcare and medications—they throw their hands up and say, "Nothing we can do about it!"

The Office of Disease Prevention and Health Promotion is one government program that I think has a lot to offer.[5] Their website is up to date, easy to navigate, has good data and some good articles on how to live a healthier life that includes *real-life* things you can do to get healthier. It helps you make a plan for your diet and activity level that is consistent with a lifestyle in the 2020s, not the early 2000s.

The problem with this useful information is its accessibility. It's only on a hidden corner of the internet. There are no advertisements about its offerings to the public. I'd never heard of this government office and program until I literally Googled "government health initiatives," so it would be great for the average American to have more access to this and have it be more well known. Also, there are many people in this country that have no access to the internet, never mind to a regular doctor's office.

So, given the sparsity of information and support from the government for us to lead a healthy life, and the absolute price-gouging that they allow to occur when it comes to the prices of healthcare in America, it's hard for me to believe that they truly have our best interests at heart. Let's be real, the prices of healthcare are not regulated because it benefits the companies' profits and the government employees who are being lobbied and bribed by these companies to not pass through any bill that will regulate prices and affect their bottom line.

And let's be even more clear here: it is not just ONE industry doing this lobbying and bribing. It is ALL of them, from the pharmaceutical industry to the insurance companies, to the equipment manufacturers, to the distributors, to the hospitals themselves. No one wants regulations placed on the amount of capital they can obtain. And let's not get started on the food industry.

Recently, I cared for a patient in the ICU—we'll call him "Marvin."

Marvin is a homeless man who lives on the streets in my

town. He has a chronic injury from a past accident that causes him constant pain, and he self-medicates with a combination of methamphetamine, heroin, marijuana, and narcotic pills. He also has type 1 diabetes, a condition that requires strict medical management. Unfortunately, Marvin frequently arrives in our emergency department in a life-threatening state of diabetic ketoacidosis (DKA), where dangerously high blood sugars cause the body to begin shutting down.

When Marvin comes in, the pattern is always the same. He's often confused, combative, and in physical distress. We typically start him on an insulin drip and admit him to the ICU. He receives pain management, Suboxone to ease withdrawal symptoms, and continuous monitoring. Despite our efforts, he often refuses treatment, becomes aggressive with staff, and leaves the hospital against medical advice—sometimes after removing his IVs or medical devices.

During his most recent visit, Marvin was severely disoriented. He shouted at staff, resisted care, and was unable to walk safely on his own. For his protection—and ours—we had to place soft limb restraints on him and administer mild sedation. Overnight, the insulin and IV fluids began to stabilize his condition.

When I arrived the next morning, I could hear him yelling profanities from down the hall. It was a challenging start to the shift. Later, while attempting to provide basic hygiene care, he became aggressive with me. He spit at me, kicked me in the stomach, and made a disturbing comment that was a threat of sexual violence.

As healthcare professionals, we are trained to separate behavior caused by illness or intoxication from intentional harm. Still, moments like this are traumatizing. I did everything I could to protect myself and maintain professionalism, but the emotional toll lingers.

What was most difficult to accept, though, was the knowledge that Marvin's entire hospital stay, including days in the ICU, medications, interventions, and staffing, was likely to be written off entirely. If he was covered by Medicaid, reimbursement would be minimal. If not, the hospital would absorb the entire cost. Either way, Marvin would not be financially responsible for his care.

This is where I struggle—not with Marvin as a person, but with the broken system that enables endless cycles of crisis without accountability or long-term solutions. Marvin's hospitalizations are frequent, expensive, and typically ineffective. He leaves before receiving the full benefit of treatment, only to return in worse shape weeks or months later.

Multiply this scenario across the country, and it's easy to see how costs compound.

Meanwhile, if someone like me—a nurse with full-time employment and private insurance—were hospitalized for DKA, I would likely face thousands of dollars in medical bills, even with coverage. I'd be financially penalized for becoming seriously ill, while someone like Marvin receives full care, regardless of outcome, at no personal cost.

This imbalance is deeply frustrating. Not because Marvin doesn't deserve care, but because the system makes it harder for working individuals to afford help while pouring resources into chronic, revolving-door cases without support structures to break the cycle. We need a healthcare system that doesn't punish people for working and paying into it. But we also need compassionate, structured approaches to address homelessness, mental health, addiction, and chronic illness—so that people like Marvin have a path forward, not just to another ICU bed.

Insurance companies are an enormous source of suffering for the public in America. They are known for denying all kinds of life-sustaining treatments, including cancer treatment, life-saving medications for things like seizures in children, or diabetes treatments, supplies, and medications. The unfortunate thing about these denials, is that they very rarely if ever come with an explanation, they are just "denied."

The upper administration and C-suite-level people in these companies are pulling in tens of millions of dollars a year in salary. Meanwhile, the average American's life can literally be ruined or *ended* by lack of medical coverage from these predatory giants. People are starting to be aware of this disparity and it's becoming more and more of a problem.

As I mentioned in Chapter 7, I have witnessed many doctors order tests or interventions that they willingly admit the patient doesn't need, just so the one they *do* need gets covered by health insurance. There is also added pressure on doctors and medical professionals because if the wrong diagnosis code is used for a patient, their entire claim for coverage could be denied. Claims denials place much undue hardship on patients who are most likely struggling with scary health issues already.

Insurance companies have a whole playbook of ways to deny your claim and continue to focus on profits over your health (sound familiar?)

For example:

- They'll deny a claim if you used an out-of-network provider—even if it was an emergency.
- They'll insist on preauthorization for treatments or medications, making your doctor's office jump through endless hoops just to get paid.
- They'll reject claims over simple clerical errors.
- They'll exclude entire categories of care, like fertility treatments, so you end up paying out-of-pocket despite having insurance.

- And don't forget the time limits—if you or your provider file too late, they'll deny your claim, no questions asked.

These denials place financial pressure and emotional stress on patients and their families, and they can delay critically needed time-sensitive care. I probably would have taken my son to the Children's Hospital emergency room way before I did if I hadn't been so scared of the cost.

There are ways to appeal a denial decision, but appeals are generally very time consuming and don't have high success rates. In an article on propublica.org titled *How Cigna Saves Millions by Having its Doctors Reject Claims Without Reading Them*, the authors investigate how insurance companies are using algorithms to systematically deny claims without actually reviewing the case.[6]

Who exactly is holding these companies accountable for their actions?

There are several governing bodies that claim to keep health insurance companies in line, including state insurance departments, the Centers for Medicare and Medicaid Services, the Department of Labor, Consumer Protection Agencies, and nonprofit advocacy groups. The problem with these agencies is that any "help" is usually retroactive.

In other words, your claim is denied, and all you can do now is file an appeal or report your insurance company to one of these entities. But in the meantime, what are you supposed to do as a patient that requires these treatments or medications to sustain your life? In some cases, there may be a workaround of some kind, but in most there is not.

The complicated nature of our system in America should not put people's lives or health at risk. We need to streamline the insurance billing process to make it the same across insurance companies, and to reduce the denials to some but not to others. We need to put our focus back on the overall health of our public, and not on the bottom lines of these enormous insurance companies.

Health insurance in America was created to offer protection; it was developed as a security in times of crisis. But for far too many, it's become a source of fear and confusion. I've lived this reality as both a nurse and a mother.

I've watched my son struggle to breathe, only to be met with a bill so large it took me six years to pay it off. I've seen patients like Marvin cycle through hospitals, costing the system tens of thousands of dollars each year, with no long-term solution in place for his health or for the burden placed on the system. Meanwhile, working families like mine pour money into monthly premiums, only to be denied, overbilled, or left footing the bill for care that should be covered.

Behind every denial letter is a child who didn't get medication, a patient with delayed care, or a family overwhelmed with debt.

Behind every inflated bill is an insurance company deciding which lives are worth saving—and how much that life is worth.

The system isn't broken by accident; it was built this way. And until we stop protecting profits over people, until we stop allowing insurers to dictate care from behind corporate desks, we will keep watching patients fall through the cracks of a system that claims to serve them.

We deserve better. We deserve coverage that actually *covers*, and care that doesn't come at the cost of everything else.

CHAPTER 11

HEALTH AS REBELLION

HEALING OURSELVES, HEALING THE SYSTEM

WE LIVE in a world where our health is too often exchanged for convenience, comfort, and the illusion of control. We trade long-term well-being for short-term ease, often without realizing how steep the cost can be—or that we may never fully get it back. We've been conditioned to hand over our autonomy to systems that profit from our sickness. But if we're willing to pause, reflect, and act, we can uncover a deeper truth: reclaiming our health is not just possible—it's essential.

This chapter isn't about blame or shame. It's about understanding the forces that keep us stuck—and rediscovering the power each of us holds to shift our own trajectory. It is about what we as individuals can do to get and keep ourselves out of this broken healthcare system, and not become forever patients.

While systemic reform is urgently needed, it will take time. So, the question becomes: *what do we do in the meantime?*

The answer begins with us. There are meaningful, empowering actions we can take right now to reduce our dependence on a broken system, improve our quality of life, and protect our future.

Our physical and mental health should be our most valued assets. Yet far too often, they're pushed aside in favor of comfort, convenience, or instant gratification. When we begin to see that our health is primarily *our* responsibility—not the government's, not the healthcare system, and not even our doctor's—we start to take back control. Today's healthcare industry focuses on treating illness, not preventing it. It manages symptoms instead of healing root causes. It prioritizes profit over people.

And while we fight for that to change, we must also protect ourselves from within.

If more of us took proactive ownership of our health, we could shift the system's burden from chronic illness to acute and unavoidable care. We'd be less reliant on prescription medications, less vulnerable to insurance loopholes, and more resilient as individuals and communities.

Of course, this kind of transformation is easier said than done. Change takes courage, energy, and persistence. Human nature is a paradox—we are capable of astonishing adaptation and progress, yet we're often paralyzed by fear, habit, and doubt. Even lifesaving change can feel impossible when we're overwhelmed.

As a nurse, I've witnessed firsthand how deeply people can resist change—even when their lives depend on it. I've had patients sit across from me and say, almost defiantly, things like: *"I eat fast food every day, even though I know it's killing me."*

They say it with a shrug—sometimes with a laugh, sometimes with shame—but always with a resignation that's quietly heartbreaking.

Why do we make choices that hurt us, even when we know better? The answer is rarely simple. It's not laziness. It's not ignorance. It's fear. It's habit. And often, it's a sense of hopelessness so deeply ingrained that change feels impossible. For many, the idea of a healthier life feels like climbing a mountain without a visible summit. They tell themselves, *"I've always been this way,"* or *"It's too late for me."*

These beliefs, left unchallenged, become self-fulfilling prophecies.

Comfort, as it turns out, is one of the most powerful addictions. The routines we build—even the ones that damage us—become our refuge. Processed foods, for instance, aren't just easy—they're engineered to be addictive. Sugar, salt, and fat light up the brain's reward system, creating cravings that are biologically difficult to resist.

These foods don't just satisfy hunger; they soothe emotional pain, mask stress, and give momentary relief. But they also keep us stuck. If we want more than just survival—if we want vitality, energy, and freedom—we have to reclaim our power. We have to believe in the possibility of change again.

Physical inactivity is another deeply embedded habit—and one of the hardest to break. For someone who's never exercised regularly, even something as small as a daily walk can feel like a monumental challenge. They may fear judgment, discomfort, or failure. These unspoken anxieties create invisible walls that keep people stuck in patterns they desperately want to escape. Often, people don't avoid change because they don't care—they avoid it because they're afraid they'll fail. And failure, especially when it comes to our bodies and health, can feel deeply personal.

This fear is magnified by the images we consume daily. Social media bombards us with filtered perfection: sculpted bodies, glowing skin, effortless energy. When you're struggling just to feel well, these idealized portrayals can make the idea of change feel not just hard, but hopeless.

Why bother starting at all, when you feel like you'll never

catch up? So, many people stay stuck. Not because they don't want more, but because they're convinced they can't have it.

Breaking these cycles takes more than just willpower. It requires understanding and addressing the emotional roots beneath the behavior. If someone uses food to manage stress, the answer isn't simply "eat better"—it's to develop healthier tools to cope: therapy, mindfulness, connection, and compassion. Without treating the *why* behind the habit, the habit won't change.

And let's be honest—the sheer size of the task can feel crushing. When someone is facing obesity, high blood pressure, diabetes, or mental health struggles, the list of things they're "supposed" to fix can feel endless: eat better, move more, sleep more, stress less, quit smoking, drink less. It's overwhelming. And when you're already feeling hopeless, a mountain of expectations is enough to make anyone give up before they even begin.

Shame is a quiet but powerful force that keeps many people stuck in place. In our society, those who struggle with their weight, chronic illness, or unhealthy habits are often labeled—consciously or unconsciously—as lazy, weak, or undisciplined. These harmful narratives don't motivate change; they deepen wounds. They push people into isolation, into silence, and into self-blame.

Shame rarely leads to healing—it usually leads to hiding. This cycle is painful and persistent. People who feel judged or misunderstood may avoid doctor's visits altogether—not out of apathy, but out of fear. Fear of being scolded instead of supported. Fear of feeling like a failure in a place that's supposed to offer help. And so, they stay away, missing out on the very care that could help them heal. This emotional barrier is just as real as any physical symptom.

If we want to break that cycle, we must shift both how we

care for ourselves—and how we think about healthcare altogether. The ultimate goal is not just treatment; it's prevention. It's about catching illness before it takes hold.

If we begin to address the root causes of chronic disease, like poor nutrition, inactivity, and unmanaged stress, we can reduce the overwhelming strain on hospitals and clinics, cut costs, and dramatically improve our quality of life.

Imagine a world where health is the norm, not the exception. Where fast food is an occasional treat, not a daily necessity. Where movement is joyful and part of daily life—not something to dread.

In that world, we would need fewer medications. Fewer emergency visits. Fewer specialists. The system itself would be forced to evolve—not because it wanted to, but because we no longer fed its dysfunction.

But to get there, we need a collective shift. It starts with individual responsibility—yes—but also with deep compassion and systemic accountability. It means changing how we eat, move, and manage stress, while also demanding better from the systems around us. This isn't just about adding years to our lives; it's about adding life to our years, and offering a better, freer, healthier world for the ones who come after us.

It's human nature to feel overwhelmed when our health begins to slip. And in that overwhelm, it can be easy to fall into a victim mindset—telling ourselves things like, *"I guess I have high blood pressure now; well, there's nothing I can do about that."*

But here's the hard truth: while many factors may be outside our control, far more are within it. And the moment we realize that is the moment everything can start to change.

Blame can feel like protection. It gives us something to point to: our genetics, our schedule, our upbringing, our environment. And yes, those factors are important. They shape our challenges. But they don't have to define our future. When we surrender all responsibility, we surrender all power. And you deserve better than that. You deserve to take your health back—and to know that it's possible.

One powerful way we can begin to reclaim that control is by shifting our relationship with medication. The pharmaceutical industry thrives on dependency. But what if we started showing up to our appointments differently? What if, instead of expecting a prescription, we expected a *conversation*—about movement, food, sleep, stress, and support?

This isn't about rejecting all medications—many people need them, and some always will. It's about being intentional. Asking questions. Seeking alternatives when appropriate. If more of us began choosing lifestyle over pill bottles when possible, the industry would be forced to respond. And that shift could ripple outward—into policy, pricing, and public health.

You have the right to understand your body, to question your care, and to be an active participant in your healing. And when enough of us do that? We begin to rewrite the rules.

Of course, there will always be people who require ongoing medical care—no matter how healthy their lifestyle. Conditions like cancer, autoimmune diseases, genetic disorders, and serious infections exist, and they deserve both our compassion and our attention.

But imagine if we could eliminate even *a fraction* of the preventable hospitalizations, emergency visits, and lifelong medication dependencies that are driven by lifestyle-related illness. The ripple effect would be enormous. Fewer people suffering. Fewer resources drained. More time, energy, and funding available to care for those who truly need it.

Part of the problem is that the food and healthcare industries are not separate—they're deeply entwined. One feeds the other, literally. Our diets have become dominated by ultra-processed, chemically manipulated foods designed not to nourish us, but to hook us. As a result, we're left overfed but undernourished—chasing energy, clarity, and health in a system that is working against us.

But what if we flipped the script? What if, instead of consuming mostly processed food, we chose real, whole, nutrient-dense meals most of the time? How about making that choice even a quarter of the time? What if we stopped giving our bodies things designed in labs, and started fueling them with things grown from the earth?

It's a simple shift—but one with revolutionary potential. A healthier population would need fewer pills, fewer procedures, and fewer devices. And when that need drops, the industries that profit from our dependency are forced to change.

Listen, I've been there, I'm speaking from the middle of this fight. I've lived the extremes. I've struggled with my weight, my mental health, and my habits. I've looked in the mirror and hated what I saw. I've climbed a flight of stairs and felt my heart race and lungs burn so bad it was embarrassing. I've turned to fast food, alcohol, and self-destructive coping mechanisms more times than I can count. I've watched family members suffer, and I've cared for thousands of patients whose lives were forever altered by conditions that might have been prevented.

And on the other end, I've fallen into the trap of perfectionism. I've chased the "ideal" body to the point of obsession—taking performance-improving substances, tracking every calorie, pushing my body past the point of health in pursuit of an image that never felt like enough. I've hurt myself in the name of wellness.

But I've learned. I've stepped off that tightrope and found something better: balance. Clarity. Self-respect. I've reclaimed my health, not perfectly, and not all at once, but with persistence and compassion. And if I can do it, I truly believe others can too.

We have more power than we think.

For too long, we've been taught to hand over that power to doctors, insurance companies, the pharmaceutical industry, and the food industries that profit from our cravings and our convenience. We've been told that health is something that happens to us, not something we can actively build, protect, and reclaim.

But that narrative is not only false, it's dangerous. And it's keeping us sick.

Real change doesn't start in Washington. It starts in kitchens and grocery stores. It starts in walking shoes and water bottles. It starts in the quiet decision to cook instead of drive-thru, to stretch instead of scroll, to rest instead of self-destruct.

And it starts, most of all, with the belief that your health and your future are worth fighting for.

I'm not here to tell you it's easy. It's not. It will require discomfort. It will require rewiring habits that have brought you comfort for years. It will require you to meet yourself honestly and tenderly—without judgment, but without excuses. You will fail. You will restart. But you need to keep going, and little by little, you'll change. And that change will ripple through your family, your workplace, and your community.

That change, multiplied, is how destructive systems fall.

We don't have to wait for healthcare reform to start healing. We can begin today. With every decision to nourish instead of numb, to move instead of freeze, to speak up instead of shrink, we reclaim a little more of what was taken from us. This is how we weaken the grip of the industries that thrive on our dependence. This is how we reclaim autonomy in a system that profits from our passivity. This is how we protect our bodies, our minds, and our children's futures.

So no, this chapter isn't just about getting healthy. It's about getting *free*.

Your health is not a burden—it's your birthright. And you are not powerless.

You are the system's worst nightmare: an awake, aware, and activated human being who has chosen to fight back—by getting well.

CHAPTER 12

A BROKEN SYSTEM AND A NATION IN CRISIS

WHAT NEEDS TO HAPPEN

AS THE PREVIOUS chapters have made clear, the American healthcare system is a mess.

Whether you've worked inside it or been caught in it as a patient, the dysfunction is impossible to miss. COVID didn't just crack the system's surface—it shattered it, exposing decades of hidden fractures and festering failures. From the abuse of healthcare workers to the stranglehold of Big Pharma and insurance giants, every layer is soaked in problems.

And they hurt *everyone*.

I could go on about how broken it all is—hell, I just did by writing this book! But this isn't just a rant. This is about what we can do next.

In the previous chapter, we looked at what people can do to take control of their health and step away from a system designed to exploit them. In this final chapter, we flip the lens. This one's about what the system itself needs to do—how we rebuild, restructure, and finally, make healthcare actual *care again*.

COVID

COVID was a wake-up call—but not the kind that inspires change. It was the kind that shakes you awake in a cold sweat, leaves you panicked, and makes you want to roll over and hit snooze. The pandemic revealed a government healthcare structure that was unprepared, disorganized, and completely misaligned with the reality on the ground.

Hospitals turned into war zones. Healthcare workers faced impossible conditions: no PPE, constantly changing protocols, and a relentless wave of patients—some dying, many terrified, all desperate. The psychological toll on all of us will linger for years.

And what did most healthcare workers get in return for their heroic efforts? A few applause videos. A hospital banner calling us "heroes." Maybe a pizza party. What we didn't get were real raises, policy reform, or systems that could support us through the trauma we were asked to endure.

The monster bared its teeth: healthcare workers are essential—but expendable.

So, what do we need to do to prevent history from repeating itself?

First and foremost, we need transparency and truth. The public deserves facts, not politically motivated half-truths, manipulative messaging, and certainly not threats or censorship. We need national leaders who understand their role is not to obsessively control the message, but to elevate the voices of those in the trenches. During COVID, frontline doctors were silenced, punished, and in some cases threatened with license revocation for speaking out or trying alternative approaches. Meanwhile, the loudest voice in the room was a bureaucrat who does not seem to have a practice grounded in current reality.

If we want a different outcome next time, we need leaders who know when to step back and let experienced clinicians lead. We need to understand that the government doesn't necessarily have its fingers on the pulse of fighting diseases at the frontline level. We need political leaders who take a step back and *become the voice to the people who are in the trenches.*

They need to listen acutely and well to our doctors who have their boots on the ground, and announce their findings to the world, instead of thinking they know best and punishing someone for having a different idea than theirs.

And we need to ensure no healthcare professional is ever again punished for using their judgment to try to save lives. The silencing of dissent during the pandemic didn't just stifle innovation—it cost lives.

Fauci and his allies didn't just get it wrong—they punished people who got it *less wrong.* They doubled down on poor science. They politicized medicine. And they left a trail of distrust that we are still reeling from today. If he had truly cared about the public, he would have welcomed all ideas, promoted open dialogue, and acknowledged that no one person holds all the answers. But instead, he—and others like him—seem to have chosen power over truth.

And here's the thing: the pandemic didn't just expose the cracks in our healthcare system, it exposed just how far money is placed above human life in this country.

More people became rich during the COVID era than in the previous 14 years.[1] While people were dying, losing loved ones, and drowning in medical bills, others were getting richer by the minute, quietly, behind the curtain of public health messaging. One of the most public figureheads during this was Tony Fauci. He had a big presence in the media during the pandemic, but much of what he said publicly has since become problematic for him. He has been called out by many people for his transgressions.

In fact, he was called before a Select Subcommittee of the Committee on Oversight and Accountability (previously known as the Committee on Oversight and Government Reform) in the summer of 2024.[2] Several important things were uncovered during these sessions. One is that he seems to have absolutely no remorse for the hundreds of thousands of lives lost because of his divisive rhetoric, partisan bullshit, and arbitrary (nay, *made up*) policies like the six-foot distance rule.

Instead of acknowledging the mistakes, the contradictions, or the policies that tore families apart, he deflected. During the hearing, he admitted that the six-foot distancing guideline—something that caused social chaos, shutdowns, and emotional harm—*wasn't even based on science*. It was a guess. A placeholder.

Meanwhile, people lost jobs, friends, and trust over it. People were actually fighting in real life because of this made-up rule.

Even more troubling is his shifting position on gain-of-function (GOF) research—the controversial scientific practice that may have been linked to COVID's origin. Fauci long denied US involvement in funding GOF research, but other NIH officials have since contradicted that claim. And the so-called "lab leak theory"? Once ridiculed as a conspiracy, it is now acknowledged by Fauci himself as a real possibility.

Suddenly, the man who helped label dissenters as dangerous is keeping an "open mind." Convenient.

Then there's the matter of censorship. During the pandemic, countless voices—doctors, researchers, and everyday citizens—were silenced for questioning the official narrative. Social media companies came under government pressure to suppress posts and articles that challenged CDC or NIH talking points.

Years later, in January 2025 interview with Joe Rogan, Mark Zuckerberg himself admitted that Facebook was placed under *extreme pressure* by Biden administration government officials—"like something out of 1984"—to flag and fact-check pandemic content.[3] That's not "public health communication." That's coordinated suppression of free speech.

The biggest lesson we need to take away from this global trauma is: be careful who you trust.

When something doesn't make sense—when it smells like bullshit—it probably is. And we need to stop being afraid to call it out. From the very beginning, I knew the six-foot distancing rule was nonsense. Whether you believed at the time that COVID spread by droplets or aerosols, that number wasn't grounded in science—it was a guess. And don't even get me started on the mask mandates.

One of the most absurd things I've ever witnessed was watching people drive alone in their cars wearing a mask, or walking around with a loose bandana over their face (or typically, just mouth) like it was going to protect them from a virus. Meanwhile, real protective gear, like N95 masks, was in short supply in hospitals.

Now, don't get me wrong. I never questioned the use of proper PPE in clinical settings. Of course I wore my N95 in the hospital. But what I *did* question was the performative, fear-driven theatrics happening everywhere else. And when I tried to speak up about it at work? I was shut down. Completely. Many of my coworkers swallowed everything the CDC and Tony Fauci said without question. Hook, line, and sinker.

There was no room for dialogue—no space for critical thinking.

And that right there? *That is the problem.*

Blind trust in authority is dangerous—especially when the information coming from that authority is inconsistent, contradictory, or outright fabricated. We have to stop handing over our brains and our rights just because some rich person in a suit tells us to. We need to do our own research, think for ourselves, and have the courage to speak up—even when it's unpopular.

Especially when it's unpopular.

We need to protect our constitutional rights—not just from foreign threats, but from domestic ones. From the people and institutions who claim to serve us, but who gaslight us, shame us, and manipulate us when it serves their agenda. We cannot let fear turn us into followers who stop asking questions. We need to stop being sheep.

BURNOUT

If you thought COVID was bad, let me tell you something that many people don't realize: healthcare workers have been dealing with abuse long before the pandemic made headlines. Physical assaults. Verbal assaults. Emotional manipulation. It's disturbingly common—and it's getting worse. COVID didn't invent this abuse; it just amplified it. Suddenly, we weren't just nurses or doctors—we were scapegoats for a terrified public.

The statistics are staggering, nearly half of all nurses' report being physically assaulted at work. Even more face constant verbal abuse. Imagine waking up, putting on your scrubs, and knowing that someone might spit on you, hit you, or scream obscenities in your face today—and that *no one will do anything about it.*

And it's not just the patients. Family members can be just as cruel—demanding unrealistic care, lashing out when expectations aren't met, or throwing tantrums because the system didn't cater to them fast enough. We're expected to handle it with grace and professionalism. But behind that calm face is someone breaking.

Most of the time, we're told to "suck it up." To be the bigger person. Administrators shrug off the abuse as "part of the job," leaving us to fend for ourselves. No protection. No backup. Just a toxic culture that normalizes cruelty in the name of customer service.

And this toxic culture is destroying us. It's driving good people out of the profession in droves. Burnout is everywhere, and it's not because we're weak—it's because the system is. Long hours. Inadequate pay. Repeated exposure to trauma with no support. Chronic understaffing. Endless bureaucratic red tape. These aren't minor inconveniences; they're soul-crushers.

Burnout doesn't just harm healthcare workers—it puts patients at risk. Exhausted, overwhelmed staff are more likely to make mistakes. And those mistakes can cost lives. But what do we get in response? A poster in the break room about resilience. A five-minute meditation app. Maybe a free coffee on "appreciation day."

It's insulting. It's performative. And it completely misses the point. Burnout is not a personal failure—it's a systemic one. And until we address the root causes, we'll keep watching some of the most passionate, skilled, and caring people walk away from the field for good.

How can we fix the burnout problem as a nation?

Well, the first thing is to radically change the culture of bedside healthcare. It should *NEVER* be acceptable, under any circumstances, to assault a healthcare worker. There need to be more federal level laws that protect us. Administration should start to have their employee's backs more than making excuses for shitty patient and family behavior. Verbal, mental, and emotional abuse should not ever be tolerated for any reason in healthcare.

The moment someone gets verbally aggressive, shouts, or is degrading in any way to a healthcare worker, that employee should be removed from their service as a protection for the EMPLOYEE. If the patient is hostile to everyone on the unit and there are no further caregivers for them, then hospitals should be able to release, discharge, and fire patients. Patients know that hospitals can't kick them out, so the shitty ones act even worse.

We need to categorically have healthcare workers backs and concentrate more on protecting them than the customer service star ratings of the hospital or company.

Second, we need nationwide mandatory staffing ratios—not just in hospitals, but in every area of healthcare. There are never enough staff *anywhere,* not in doctor's offices, long-term care facilities, assisted living centers, home health, hospice, urgent care—you name it. There is a chronic, dangerous lack of staff in nearly every corner of this industry. And it's breaking people.

California has shown that union-enforced nurse-to-patient ratios save lives and reduce burnout.[4] So why aren't we doing this everywhere? Legislation must be passed to prevent healthcare facilities from taking on new patients if they don't have enough staff to safely care for the ones they already have. It's common sense—and a matter of safety.

We also need more flexible scheduling models. Not everyone can sustain twelve-hour shifts every week of the year. Why not offer alternative options like eight-hour rotations, four-hour overlaps, or shift-sharing models that allow for better work-life balance?

These aren't radical ideas—they're *basic retention strate-*

gies. We can't solve burnout if we keep designing systems that burn people out by default.

Finally, we need to treat the emotional toll of this work as the legitimate psychological trauma that it is. Healthcare workers witness pain, suffering, death, and human despair on a regular basis. Most people would need therapy after watching one traumatic event. Healthcare workers witness dozens—sometimes hundreds—throughout their careers. And many do it without support.

Every healthcare institution in this country should have access to free, on-site or partnered mental health services for their staff. At the very least, because of the work we do, employees should be offered free sessions with a licensed therapist or psychiatrist. For smaller organizations, partnerships with local providers could make this feasible without enormous overhead. Even peer-to-peer support groups or a designated space to decompress and connect could make a meaningful difference. We talk a lot about "resilience" in this field—but resilience doesn't come from being left alone to suffer. It comes from being *seen, heard, and supported.*

The culture of healthcare is to just internally suffer, not really talk about it, and be "tough." Well, that only lasts for so long until even the strongest person breaks. The solutions are not out of reach. But they require leadership with the courage to value people over profit—and to treat healthcare workers like the essential humans they are.

DOCTORS

The image of the respected, independent physician has been replaced by a new reality: endless paperwork, crushing student debt, and a system that prioritizes profits over patients. Doctors are increasingly being squeezed by insurance companies, Big

Pharma, and hospital administrators who care more about the bottom line than quality of care.

Many doctors are leaving private practice altogether, opting for salaried positions that offer a semblance of stability but come with their own set of challenges. Others are leaving the profession entirely, burned out by a system that demands more than it gives. And who can blame them? It's hard to focus on patient care when you're drowning in bureaucracy and battling insurance companies over every little thing.

How can we fix the system for doctors?

My first idea is that the US adopts a nation-wide electronic medical record (EMR) system. There are several countries across the world that have done this—including Estonia, Sweden, Denmark, and Singapore—and it streamlines patient care and decreases administrative burden on doctors and their office staff.[5]

Basically, there is one single database and medical record for each registered citizen of these countries. This way, any doctor across the entire country has access to the entirety of each patient's medical records, and as they are updated, their other providers have real-time access to the new records.

In the US, we have a fractured system of competing EMRs that *don't talk to each other*. This creates dangerous gaps in care and wastes time, money, and energy. One specialist has no idea what another is doing. Lab results fall through the cracks. Medications get duplicated.

It's not just inefficient—it's dangerous. We either need one unified national EMR, or we need to force interoperability between all existing EMR systems through a centralized data hub. Every provider, regardless of software platform, should have access to patient records when it counts. This would reduce overhead, improve care coordination, and lower long-term healthcare costs by cutting waste and improving outcomes.

Another idea for helping doctors out is reforming the insurance reimbursement process. Prior authorizations are the bane of doctor's existences. They cannot do their jobs because the intervention they are trying to use for the patient must go through 47 different people and areas of the insurance companies to get "prior authorization." And then sometimes, even with this, they are still denied payment. This increases burnout, stress, and frustration in doctors because they are forced to deal with a mountain of paperwork and documentation for each of their patients, and they are taken away from patient care to deal with these convoluted systems.

Reimbursement rates for general primary care doctors are *FAR* less than surgeons or specialists. This has led to a shortage of primary care physicians because who would want to be the low man on the totem pole? Reimbursement should be fairer across the board. Getting reimbursed for care should not be as difficult as it is.

Streamlining these processes by simplifying the insurance companies' systems would greatly decrease the burden held by doctors. If the patient has an established chronic illness diagnosis, then NO intervention for this diagnosis should require prior authorization. Prior authorization should be reserved for experimental, extremely expensive, or non-FDA approved interventions. Having to prior-authorize someone's blood pressure medication is literal insanity. Doctors should be allowed to focus on medicine—not memorizing insurance loopholes. We need our physicians back at the bedside—not buried in billing software.

BIG PHARMA AND BIG INSURANCE

Let's not beat around the bush: Big Pharma and insurance companies are two of the biggest culprits in the downfall of American healthcare.

Drug prices are astronomical, and insurance coverage is a labyrinth of confusion and inequity. Patients are forced to choose between paying their rent and buying life-saving medications. Meanwhile, insurance companies rake in billions while denying claims and dictating what treatments patients can and can't receive.

The relationship between Big Pharma, insurance companies, and the government is deeply problematic. Lobbyists wield immense power, shaping policies that benefit corporations at the expense of everyday Americans. The result is a healthcare system that's driven by profit, not patient outcomes. It's a system where money talks and the most vulnerable are left to fend for themselves.

This is not a healthcare system. It's a profit machine.

The astronomical cost of prescription medications in the United States is a glaring problem. Drugs that are lifesaving for some are priced so exorbitantly that many patients are forced to ration their medications or forgo them entirely, often with devastating consequences.

Capping drug prices would ensure that essential medications are accessible to everyone, not just those who can afford them. Transparency in pricing is equally crucial. Far too often, patients and even healthcare providers are kept in the dark about the true cost of medications, leading to surprise bills and financial strain.

When pharmaceutical companies use public funds for research, they should not be allowed to price-gouge the public for the final product. If taxpayer dollars helped develop it, then the public should have affordable access to it. And yes, Medicare must be allowed to negotiate with pharmaceutical companies. Allowing Medicare to negotiate would immediately decrease drug prices. This would put the power back in the government's hands when it comes to the price of medications, which is important, because our government frequently funds the research and development of these drugs.

Then there's patent abuse, like "evergreening" (see page 197). This makes the market less competitive because generic drugs are kept off the market sometimes for decades, which drives up medication prices and lines the pockets of Big Pharma companies. It's legal manipulation, and it should be illegal.

For life-sustaining, irreplaceable treatments medications like insulin, there should be price caps and zero patents. These drugs should be readily available, accessible, and affordable to anyone who needs them. No exceptions. No profit-driven delay. In fact, the original developers of insulin did not patent it for this exact reason.

And let me be clear: I say all of this as someone who generally supports *less* government regulation. But this is different. This is life and death. The pharmaceutical industry has proven it will not regulate itself.

Every time reform is proposed, Big Pharma spends billions lobbying politicians into silence. They don't even hide it anymore. They don't have to. There should be strict limitations placed on pharmaceutical lobbying and campaign donations.

Also, if a government employee obtains money from a Big Pharma company, this should be public knowledge-we should be able to see the amount of times money was given to each politician and how much. This would show instantly the politicians who are prioritizing lining their pockets over people's LIVES. Pressure from the public on making these lobby deals more transparent is a must. We have a right to know who's being bought—and at what cost. Because when politicians are making decisions that affect our health, we deserve to know whether they're protecting *people* or *profits*.

Insurance companies, on the other hand, must be held accountable for their role in creating an empire of red tape, confusion, and financial fear. Prior authorizations, denials of medically necessary treatment, and skyrocketing premiums create an exhausting system where patients must constantly fight just to get basic care. Every American has a horror story. We all know what it feels like to suffer at the hands of an insurance company—and we're told that's just the way it is.

It doesn't have to be.

UNIVERSAL HEALTHCARE

The US insurance industry is a dumpster fire—and it's hard to fix something this complex and corrupted. I've spent *many hours* researching possible solutions, and I've experienced this nightmare firsthand. So have you. So has nearly everyone you know. And whenever I talk about solutions, someone inevitably says, "Well, what about free healthcare?"

Let's dive into this as a possibility for the US.

Universal healthcare. Free healthcare for all.

It sounds idyllic and wonderful. From the outside, it sounds like a no brainer, and it's difficult to understand why we don't have it in this country.

According to the WHO, Universal Healthcare (UHC) is a type of healthcare that grants all citizens of a country the full range of health services they need, when they need it, and where they need it without financial hardship.[6] It should cover all aspects of healthcare from preventative medicine to treatment of illnesses to palliative care at end of life.

There are several benefits of UHC, and they benefit the patient, not businesses. The most important one, in my opinion, is the increase in positive health outcomes for our people. UHC allows people to obtain the medical treatment they need without any concern of the cost, so people would likely be much more willing to go to the doctor multiple times a year to maintain their health. They would be more willing to go to urgent care or the hospital if they feel it's necessary without putting it off until it's too late.

I am certain that it would increase preventative medicine visits which could only result in a net positive. There will always be people who do not seek health care until it's too late, but for the majority of people it would improve total outcomes and save money by reducing the need for expensive emergency treatment and long-term disease management.

Another huge benefit of UHC systems is that they create health equity.

Right now in America, healthcare access is determined by income, employment status, and zip code. It's a caste system, plain and simple. The wealthy get cutting-edge treatments. The poor get ER visits and debt. But under UHC, healthcare is no longer a privilege—it's a right. Everyone, regardless of socioeconomic status, has access to the same standard of care. That means chronic illness management, cancer screenings, prenatal visits, therapy—everything—would be available to all, not just the insured and the fortunate.

There are economic benefits too. If employers no longer had to provide private insurance plans, companies could save tens of millions of dollars per year. That savings could be redirected to wages, hiring, infrastructure, or innovation. Workers would be more free to change jobs without losing coverage. Families would no longer fear financial ruin because of a single medical emergency. And Americans could finally stop drowning in surprise bills, denials, and deductibles. The economic benefits for our US citizens would truly make an impact in our daily lives.

So, the big question is: *how do we pay for it?*

Technically, the answer is simple: we fund it the same way we fund public schools, highways, and defense—through taxes. But unlike our current insurance model, where we pay premiums to private companies that pocket a large portion of that money, UHC systems centralize healthcare spending and prioritize public well-being. Every dollar is tracked, every category scrutinized. Healthcare spending becomes a national budget item—just like infrastructure, defense, or education.

I think many of us consider the United Kingdom (UK) to be reasonably similar to the US in many respects, so I am going to use their universal healthcare system as a basis for explanations and examples.

The UK's UHC system is the National Health Service (NHS). This was established in 1948 after the Second World War to further support its war-fatigued citizens by providing free healthcare for everyone regardless of their income or ability to pay. About 80% of the funding for this comes from income tax on its citizens, and the rest comes mostly from what's called the National Income Contributions (NIC). These NICs are comparable to social security tax here in the US. It's a tax on top of their income taxes that goes directly to funding their healthcare system.[7]

Table 2 is a chart I put together on the taxation of UK vs US citizens:[8,9,10]

Now here's the thing.

Americans are constantly told that UHC would mean outrageous taxes. We're led to believe that our system—flawed as it may be—is still the "freedom-friendly" option. But when I look at the actual data, I disagree. I have found that there is room to tax our citizens more but still be an overall financial benefit for most people.

Category	UK	US
Income Tax (Basic Rate)	20% (on £12,571–£50,270)	12% (on $11,001–$44,725)
Income Tax (Higher Rate)	40% (on £50,271–£125,140)	24% (on $95,376–$182,100)
Income Tax (Top Rate)	45% (over £125,140)	37% (over $578,125)
Social Security / National Insurance Tax	Employees: 12% (on £12,571–£50,270), 2% (above); Employers: 13.8% (above £9,100)	Employees: 6.2% SS (up to $160,200), 1.45% Medicare; Additional 0.9% over $200,000
Sales/Consumption Tax	20% VAT (nationwide)	0%–9.5% (varies by state/locality)
Property Tax	Varies by local council and property value bands	0.5%–2% of assessed property value (varies by location)
Healthcare Spending per Capita (2022)	£3,047 (approx. $3,500)	$12,555.00
Total Tax Revenue (% of GDP)	33.5%	27.7%

Table 2 A comparison of US and UK taxes. *(As of March 2025, the UK pound (£) = $1.29).*

Although the actual percentage of taxation is higher in a place with universal health care, the annual expenditure on healthcare per household is almost four times higher in the US. This puts unnecessary financial strain on Americans. We can clearly see this, as the number one reason for filing bankruptcy in America is healthcare debt.[11]

Why? Because instead of pooling our money into a government-run healthcare system that covers everyone, we funnel it into for-profit private insurance companies and pharmaceutical companies who charge astronomical premiums, deny coverage, and still leave millions of Americans with crushing debt.

Even people with "good" insurance end up owing thousands after a major health crisis.

We are told to fear higher taxes. But the truth is, we're already paying more—we just don't get what we pay for. Our premiums, deductibles, and out-of-pocket expenses are draining families dry. And unlike taxes, those payments don't come with any guarantee of care.

Universal healthcare could change that. It could save homes, savings accounts, and futures. And for many Americans, it could finally mean freedom from the fear that getting sick = going broke.

Let's be honest—implementing universal healthcare in the US would be a massive undertaking. Unfortunately for us, we are deeply embedded on multiple levels into the private insurance industry. It will be very difficult for us to crawl our way out of this hole we have dug ourselves, and there are plenty of government officials who won't go quietly. When you've been funded and lobbied by private insurers for decades, change threatens your paycheck, not just your platform.

And then there's the biggest hurdle of all: cost.

The numbers are intimidating. The closest idea our government has had to having a UHC is that of the Medicare for All Act. This system is thought to lead to a 13% healthcare savings in the long term by providing Medicare-like benefits to all citizens regardless of income.[12]

This would be fantastic, but the cost of starting the program was estimated to be $2.4–2.8 trillion each year for at least the first ten years after implementation.[13] For 2025, the United States is projecting a TOTAL budget spending of $1.9 trillion.[14] So, the estimated cost of starting a UHC is more than our defense and non-defense budgets combined for the entire year.

Even with a shift in tax revenue and reduced private spending, these numbers are hard for lawmakers to swallow—especially in a political system already drowning in debt and dysfunction. We also need to look at the fact that the US spends way more than it makes every year already, hence our astronomical national debt of $36 trillion.[15] We need to get that spending under control, decrease our overall debt, and then perhaps we could convince some politicians to go for a UHC investment.

But historically, financial discipline isn't exactly our strong suit.

Another common argument against UHC is the idea that it will stifle medical innovation. America is known for pushing the boundaries in science and technology. The fear is that if the government controls too much of the healthcare system, profit margins will shrink and private companies will lose the incentive to innovate. And there's some truth to this concern, as it's known that Medicare as it stands today does not help innovation in itself, as its reimbursement is confusing, changing frequently, and is unpredictable.[16] Because of this, inventors and companies are never entirely sure what will be big money makers on the Medicare side of things. The thought is if "Medicare for All" were to become a thing, the issue would be exacerbated, and innovation would take a steep decline.

But here's the other side of that coin: Government-funded innovation already exists—and it works.

Take the National Institutes of Health (NIH). It's one of the largest funders of medical research in the world—and it's fully government-backed. Its work has led to breakthroughs in cancer treatment, vaccines, gene therapy, and more. So yes, we can innovate *and* regulate—if we're willing to prioritize long-term public health over short-term private gain.

That said, the transition to UHC will absolutely impact profit-driven healthcare sectors. The financial gain of these independent pharmaceutical companies, medical device companies, and private corporations like hospital chains or other sectors of the healthcare system isn't ONLY about research and development. It's about manufacturing, marketing, research and development, and profits.[17]

If the government starts negotiating every price, from gauze pads to MRI machines, it's going to hit some bottom lines hard.

Will it disrupt the current landscape?

Absolutely.

Will some companies tighten their belts or change their strategy?

Yes.

Will that hurt medical progress?

Only if we let it.

Innovation doesn't have to die under universal healthcare—but greed might. And that's exactly the point because greed over human lives needs to end.

The last major argument against UHC that I have heard over the years is that of the increased wait times and possible *worse* health outcomes.

As stated above, I have always believed that one of the overall net benefits of a UHC would be that of *improved* outcomes, but I digress. I have personally heard horror stories from Canadians who have basically fled their universal healthcare to come to America so they don't have to wait so long for desperately needed surgery or treatments. For example, Canadians sometimes have to wait up to 29 weeks to see an orthopedic specialist, so this makes something as commonplace as a knee replacement a huge ordeal there.

But here is the thing: not all universal healthcare systems are built the same.

Countries like Germany, Switzerland, and Australia have universal coverage without the long wait times. Why? Because they run hybrid models. Citizens can choose public coverage or purchase private insurance for faster access or additional services.[18] This dual structure keeps wait times competitive, preserves innovation, and ensures no one goes without care—even if they can't afford private coverage.

So yes, let's learn from the weaknesses in other systems. But let's also stop pretending the US is some shining beacon of efficiency or excellence. Because when it comes to health outcomes, we are not leading, *we are failing*.

Let's look at the data:

- The US has the worst overall health outcomes of any high-income country.
- Our life expectancy is falling—for the first time in decades.
- We have more chronic illness, more mental health disorders, and higher suicide rates than our peers.
- We spend nearly 18% of our GDP on healthcare—almost double what other wealthy countries spend.
- Our rate of avoidable deaths (deaths that could have been prevented with basic medical care) is higher than the UK and Switzerland combined.
- Our infant mortality rate is embarrassingly high.
- Twice as many American women die during childbirth than in any other developed country.
- We are one of the most obese populations in the world—and yet somehow, we also have some of the fewest doctor visits per person.

- Despite all of this, we have fewer hospital beds per capita than most other developed countries.[19]

We as a nation are paying the most and getting the least.

So, when someone says, "Universal healthcare might make things worse," or "Universal healthcare will bankrupt our country," I have to laugh—*how could it possibly get worse than this?*

The fearmongering around UHC distracts us from the real issue: our current system is broken. People are dying, going bankrupt, and suffering in silence—not because they're lazy, not because they're irresponsible, but because our system puts profit over people, every single time.

It's time to stop defending a healthcare model that fails on every major metric.

It's time to stop pretending the status quo is acceptable.

It's time to demand something better.

I'll be honest with you.

Before I started writing this book, I was firmly in the "universal healthcare is a scam" camp. I believed that more government control almost always meant more inefficiency, more red tape, and more opportunities for corruption. I thought capitalism, flawed as it was, was still the best path forward. Let innovation thrive. Let competition sort the strong from the weak.

But then I started looking closer.

I started researching. Listening. Witnessing.

And I realized that the system I was defending wasn't just broken—it was *breaking people.*

The deeper I went, the more undeniable it became: we need major reform. We need a system that centers health, not wealth. We need a model that treats healthcare as a human right, not a luxury reserved for the fortunate. And yes, I still believe private insurance should remain an option for those who want it. But baseline access to care should be guaranteed to every single American, without exception.

When I look at the data, and compare it to what I've seen firsthand on the front lines, I can't help but feel disgusted by our current trajectory. The stats are nauseating. The suffering is everywhere. And worst of all, it's preventable. I used to think universal healthcare was a pipe dream.

Now I think it might be the only way forward.

A CASE IN POINT

I want to wrap this up with something deeply personal—because this is where it really hits home.

I've seen so much suffering in my career. So many people lost in a system that was supposed to help them but didn't. I've watched patients fall through the cracks, get buried in bureaucracy, misled by bad information, or pushed into treatments they never should've had. I've participated—unwillingly—in interventions that made me feel complicit in a system that profits from vulnerability. And I've seen hundreds of cases where I believe patients were exploited under the guise of "care."

A 2017 study published in *Health Affairs* found that *up to 30% of healthcare spending in the US may be unnecessary*, including overtreatment, redundant testing, and services that provide minimal or no clinical benefit.[20] That's three out of ten.

And honestly? I think it's higher.

Here's one case I witnessed that has stuck with me:

A patient—78 years old, with 22 separate medical diagnoses. Active smoker for 60 years. Organ systems in decline—lungs, heart, kidneys, liver. Their circulation was poor, unsurprisingly, and they were referred to a vascular surgeon.

Without hesitation, the surgeon recommended extensive

vein grafts and vascular surgery to repair 95% blocked veins in her legs.

There was no meaningful discussion of the risks. No exploration of the patient's current or future quality of life. No honest assessment of whether this patient—frail, chronically ill, and living alone—could even survive the recovery. Just: "We'll fix you right up."

The patient barely left their house. They lived alone, smoked a pack a day, and suffered from severe chronic pain (not even related to the circulation issues). They had made choices for their entire life that led up to situation they find themselves in now with essentially no accountability by medical professionals or themselves.

And yet this surgeon pitched the procedure as if it were minor and an easy fix.

There are several problems here. The first is that, in my opinion, the surgeon was lying to the patient.

This surgery, for a very chronically ill, weak, and impaired patient is *not* going to be easy for them. If it was a generally healthy 50-year-old, this statement may be true. But the truth is, no surgery for a patient in this one's condition is going to be easy.

The second is that no discussion was had about the ongoing medical issues the patient will have, and what the long-term effects of having this surgery could be, not the least of which is being placed on an anticoagulant (blood thinner) likely for the rest of their life, which can cause complications in and of itself. The chances that this patient gets an infection are incredibly high given all of their comorbidities, which increases their chances of having a prolonged hospital stay or being re-hospitalized after going home.

No discussion was had regarding the fact that this problem can also reoccur despite surgery and require a second or third surgery afterward. This patient is very medically frail, at least one of these complications is bound to happen to them.

When I spoke with them, they looked at me, confused and afraid, and said, "The surgeon made it sound like it's literally no big deal. I don't understand why they wouldn't tell me all of this."

Yeah. I don't understand either.

But that's the problem. Too often in American medicine, we treat the disease—not the person. We slice, prescribe, and intervene without truly evaluating whether the intervention makes sense for the individual. If this patient had been told the whole truth about the risks, the recovery, the impact of their smoking, and the potential for recurrence, it's most likely they would not have consented. We are legally supposed to ensure patients get enough information so they can give consent after being well informed of all aspects of the intervention. In my experience, patients are *very rarely* given the whole picture necessary to make this possible.

But fear is a powerful motivator. The surgeon warned, "If we don't do this, your leg could turn gangrenous and need amputation."

That was enough. The patient agreed—not out of confidence, but out of panic.

This isn't about demonizing specialists or doctors. Specialized docs save lives every day. But hyper-specialization without holistic insight can do harm. We have doctors in this country who specialize in the three tiny bones in your ear, and yes, that has its place. But what we desperately need more of are providers who see the whole patient. Who treat root causes, not just symptoms. Who ask: "Will this make this person's life better—or just longer and harder?"

In my opinion, that patient should never have been cleared for surgery—not while still smoking, not without changing their lifestyle at all, and not with their prognosis and comorbidities. It's not about punishment. It's about practicality, ethics, and risk. When a body is barely holding on, cutting into it for a marginal gain is not healing—it's gambling for the sake of money.

We have to understand that with every pill, every procedure, and every intervention, we are disrupting the body's natural equilibrium. And we've created a system that throws pharmaceutical and surgical band-aids on people who actually need support, education, and a different way of living.

We have to stop chasing numbers on charts and start seeing human beings.

Because three out of ten interventions being unnecessary is far too many.

LOOKING AHEAD

We are standing at a precipice. Our healthcare system isn't just cracked—it's collapsing under the weight of greed, indifference, and betrayal. We've watched it fail our patients, our families, ourselves—and worst of all, it's failing the very people still holding it up: our nurses, doctors, techs, aides, first responders, and every exhausted soul who walks into chaos every day just to try and do some good.

If we don't demand change now, then when? If we don't protect those who protect and heal us, then who will?

We can no longer accept a system that profits from pain and dares to call it progress, or policies that silence truth, punish integrity, and value corporate margins over human lives. We need reform that is bold, uncompromising, and rooted in humanity. We need to stop being sheep.

We must ask harder questions, speak louder truths, and refuse to settle for a healthcare system that treats people like numbers and suffering like revenue. Every patient, every provider, every person caught in this broken machine deserves better.

We deserve a system that heals—not one that profits off our pain.

Here's the part they never expected: we're not powerless. We can fight back—not just in Washington, but at our dinner tables, in our hospitals, in our communities, and inside ourselves. We can choose to take better care of our bodies, not because the system deserves it, but because we do. We can vote for leaders who don't take Big Pharma money, who stand up to insurance giants, who believe healthcare is a right. We can speak out, show up, and refuse to be gaslit into believing this is the best we can do.

Hope is not naive. Hope is defiant. Hope is what made me write this book. It lives in every healthcare worker who still shows up, every patient who advocates for themselves and others, every citizen who dares to believe we can do better.

We can demand reform. We can design new models. We can refuse to accept suffering as the cost of doing business.

It will take courage, unity, and relentless, unapologetic advocacy. But I believe change isn't just possible—it's inevitable. Because once enough people rise up and say, "This is not good enough," the system will have no choice but to change.

The system may be broken. But we are not.

We are brave.

NOTES

1. FEAR AND RESILIENCE

1. Gamio L, Lutz E, Sun A. As emergency ends, a look at Covid's U.S. death toll. *The New York Times.* Published May 11, 2023. https://www.nytimes.com/interactive/2023/05/11/us/covid-deaths-us.html
2. Bentley E, Stamm S, Kamp J. *The Wall Street Journal.* 2022 [cited 2025 May 29]. U.S. Surpasses One Million Covid-19 Deaths. Available from: https://www.wsj.com/health/healthcare/u-s-nears-one-million-covid-19-deaths-11650838998
3. Berche P. Life and Death of Smallpox. La Presse Médicale 2022;51(3). doi:https://doi.org/10.1016/j.lpm.2022.104117
4. National Archives and Records Administration. The Influenza Epidemic of 1918. Archives.gov. Published 2018. Accessed October 31, 2024. https://www.archives.gov/exhibits/influenza-epidemic/
5. World Health Organization. COVID-19 deaths | WHO COVID-19 dashboard. Published October 20, 2024. Accessed November 4, 2024. https://data.who.int/dashboards/covid19/deaths
6. Worldometer. Italy. Published April 13, 2024. Accessed October 31, 2024. https://www.worldometers.info/coronavirus/country/italy/
7. Alexander C. Year of the Nurse: A Covid-19 2020 Pandemic Memoir. Caskara Press; 2021.
8. Roche D. *Newsweek.* 2021 [cited 2025 May 20]. Fauci Said Masks "Not Really Effective," Email Reveals. Available from: https://www.newsweek.com/fauci-said-masks-not-really-effective-keeping-out-virus-email-reveals-1596703
9. VEKLURY® (remdesivir) ACTT-1 Study Efficacy and Safety Data | HCP. Vekluryhcp.com. Published 2017. Accessed October 27, 2024. https://www.vekluryhcp.com/inpatient?gad_source=1&gclid=CjoKC QjwpvK4BhDUARIsADHt9sSuafgTPoXuRntDUyceUQFN2Brv7t T3AfLbiLJwtPZ8ygySl_QZ5dwaAsXlEALw_wcB&gclsrc=aw.ds
10. Wang Y, Zhang D, Du G, et al. Remdesivir in adults with severe COVID-19: a randomised, double-blind, placebo-controlled, multicentre trial. The Lancet. 2020;0(0). doi:https://doi.org/10.1016/S0140-6736(20)31022-9; Yasir M, Chetan Reddy Lankala, Pravin Panditrao Kalyankar, et al. An Updated Systematic Review on Remdesivir's Safety and Efficacy in Patients Afflicted With COVID-19. Cureus. Published online August 7, 2023. doi:https://doi.org/10.7759/cureus.43060

11. McCreary EK, Angus DC. Efficacy of Remdesivir in COVID-19. JAMA 2020;324(11):1041–1042. doi:10.1001/jama.2020.16337
12. US government buys most of world's supply of COVID-19 drug remdesivir. pharmaphorum. Published July 2020. Accessed October 27, 2024. https://pharmaphorum.com/news/us-government-buys-most-of-worlds-supply-of-covid-19-drug-remdesivir
13. Office of the Commissioner. Ivermectin and COVID-19. FDA. Published online 2024. https://www.fda.gov/consumers/consumer-updates/ivermectin-and-covid-19
14. Kory P, Meduri GU, Varon J, Iglesias J, Marik PE. Review of the emerging evidence demonstrating the efficacy of Ivermectin in the prophylaxis and treatment of COVID-19. Am J Ther 2021 Apr 22;28(3):e299–e318. doi: 10.1097/MJT.0000000000001377. Erratum in: Am J Ther 2021 Nov–Dec 01;28(6):e813. PMID: 34375047; PMCID: PMC8088823.
15. Shafiee A, Teymouri Athar MM, Kohandel Gargari O, Jafarabady K, Siahvoshi S, Mozhgani SH. Ivermectin under scrutiny: a systematic review and meta-analysis of efficacy and possible sources of controversies in COVID-19 patients. Virology Journal. 2022;19(1). doi:https://doi.org/10.1186/s12985-022-01829-8
16. Chamie JJ, Hibberd JA, Scheim DE. COVID-19 Excess Deaths in Peru's 25 States in 2020: Nationwide Trends, Confounding Factors, and Correlations with the Extent of Ivermectin Treatment by State. Cureus [Internet]. [cited 2025 May 29];15(8):e43168. Available from: https://www.ncbi.nlm.nih.gov/pmc/articles/PMC10484241/; Uttar Pradesh government says early use of Ivermectin helped to keep positivity, deaths low [Internet]. *The Indian Express*. 2021 [cited 2025 May 29]. Available from: https://indianexpress.com/article/cities/lucknow/uttar-pradesh-government-says-ivermectin-helped-to-keep-deaths-low-7311786/
17. USAFacts [Internet]. 2025 [cited 2025 May 20]. US Coronavirus vaccine tracker. Available from: https://usafacts.org/visualizations/covid-vaccine-tracker-states/
18. Andersson PA, Tinghög G, Västfjäll D. The effect of herd immunity thresholds on willingness to vaccinate. Humanit Soc Sci Commun [Internet]. 2022 Jul 18 [cited 2025 May 20];9(1):1–7. Available from: https://www.nature.com/articles/s41599-022-01257-7
19. American Hospital Association. CMS eliminates COVID-19 vaccination requirements for health care workers. Published May 31, 2023. Accessed October 31, 2024. https://www.aha.org/news/headline/2023-05-31-cms-eliminates-covid-19-vaccination-requirements-health-care-workers
20. Centers for Disease Control and Prevention. NVSS - Provisional Death Counts for COVID-19 - Executive Summary. www.cdc.gov. Published January 27, 2021. https://www.cdc.gov/nchs/covid19/mortality-overview.htm

21. Woodruff RC, Tong X, Jackson SL, Loustalot FV, Vaugan AS. Trends in National Death Rates from Heart Disease in the United States, 2010–2020 [Abstract]. Circulation 2022;146 (suppl 1). https://www.ahajournals.org/doi/10.1161/circ.146.suppl_1.985
22. National Center for Health Statistics. Leading causes of death. Centers for Disease Control and Prevention. Published May 2, 2024. Accessed October 31, 2024. https://www.cdc.gov/nchs/fastats/leading-causes-of-death.htm; Xu J, Murphy S, Kochanek K, Arias E. Mortality in the United States, 2021.; 2022. https://www.cdc.gov/nchs/data/databriefs/db456.pdf; Murphy S, Kochanek K, Xu J, Arias E. Mortality in the United States, 2020 Key Findings Data from the National Vital Statistics System.; 2021. https://www.cdc.gov/nchs/data/databriefs/db427.pdf

2. BURNOUT

1. Rotenstein LS, Brown R, Sinsky C, Linzer M. The association of work overload with burnout and intent to leave the job across the healthcare workforce during COVID-19. J Gen Intern Med 2023 Jun;38(8):1920–1927. doi: 10.1007/s11606-023-08153-z. Epub 2023 Mar 23. PMID: 36959522; PMCID: PMC10035977.
2. West CP, Dyrbye LN, Shanafelt TD. Physician burnout: contributors, consequences and solutions. J Intern Med [Internet]. 2018 Jun [cited 2025 May 20];283(6):516–29. Available from: https://onlinelibrary.wiley.com/doi/10.1111/joim.12752
3. Saunders B. Empower Work. [cited 2025 May 20]. Addressing burnout takes more than self-care. Available from: https://www.empowerwork.org/blog/addressing-burnout-takes-more-than-self-care
4. Burnout. Merriam-Webster [Internet]. [cited 2025 May 20]. Available from: https://www.merriam-webster.com/dictionary/burnout

3. BEHIND THE SCRUBS

1. Bland C, Zuckerbraun S, Lines LM, et al. Challenges Facing CAHPS Surveys and Opportunities for Modernization. Research Triangle Park (NC): RTI Press; 2022 Nov. Available from: https://www.ncbi.nlm.nih.gov/books/NBK592584/ doi: 10.3768/rtipress.2022.op.0080.2211
2. Fact Sheet: Workplace Violence and Intimidation, and the Need for a Federal Legislative Response. https://www.aha.org/system/files/media/file/2022/06/fact-sheet-workplace-violence-and-intimidation-and-the-need-for-a-federal-legislative-response.pdf
3. American Hospital Association [Internet]. 2024 [cited 2025 May 21]. At AHA Briefing, Hospital Leaders Urge Congress to Pass the Save Act and Protect Health Care Workers from Violence. Available from: https://

www.aha.org/news/headline/2024-01-30-aha-briefing-hospital-leaders-urge-congress-pass-save-act-and-protect-health-care-workers-violence

4. NURSES' PROVERBIAL PLATES

1. Allnurses.com. 1950s Nursing. Published March 19, 2005. Accessed August 2, 2024. https://allnurses.com/s-nursing-t71904/
2. Centers for Medicare & Medicaid Services. CMS' Value-Based Programs | CMS. www.cms.gov. Published 2023. https://www.cms.gov/medicare/quality/value-based-programs

5. THE COST OF CARE

1. Registered Nurses: Occupational Outlook Handbook: U.S. Bureau of Labor Statistics. bls.gov. Published November 27, 2023. https://www.bls.gov/ooh/healthcare/registered-nurses.htm
2. Registered Nurses: Occupational Outlook Handbook: U.S. Bureau of Labor Statistics. bls.gov. Published April 25, 2023. https://www.bls.gov/oes/2022/may/oes291141.htm
3. Registered Nurses. Bureau of Labor Statistics. Published April 25, 2023. https://www.bls.gov/oes/2022/may/oes291141.htm
4. DeJohn J. Salary Needed to Live Comfortably – 2024 Study. smartasset.com. Published March 19, 2024. https://smartasset.com/data-studies/salary-needed-live-comfortably-2024
5. Why Nurses Quit. Medscape. https://www.medscape.com/viewarticle/why-nurses-quit-2024a1000bza?form=fpf
6. Why Nurses Quit. Medscape. https://www.medscape.com/viewarticle/why-nurses-quit-2024a1000bza?form=fpf
7. National Nurses United. NNU report shows increased rates of workplace violence experienced by nurses | National Nurses United. www.nationalnursesunited.org. Published February 5, 2024. https://www.nationalnursesunited.org/press/nnu-report-shows-increased-rates-of-workplace-violence-experienced-by-nurses
8. Gooch K. 10 Highest-Paid Healthcare CEOs. Beckershospitalreview.com. Published May 21, 2024. Accessed October 27, 2024. https://www.beckershospitalreview.com/compensation-issues/10-highest-paid-healthcare-ceos.html

   Dyrda L. Healthcare Executive Pay Jumps 4.6%: 5 notes. Beckershospitalreview.com. Published October 17, 2024. Accessed October 27, 2024. https://www.beckershospitalreview.com/compensation-issues/healthcare-executive-pay-jumps-4-6-5-notes.html

6. THE OVERWORKED, UNDERPAID, AND INDISPENSABLE CNAS

1. Oppenheimer TH. Certified Nurse Assistant (CNA) Salary Guide. Nurse.org. 30 July 2024. Accessed 8 October 2024. https://nurse.org/education/CNA-salary/
2. Crew Member Hourly Salaries in Colorado at McDonald's. Indeed. Accessed 8 October 2024. https://www.indeed.com/cmp/McDonald's/salaries/Crew-Member/Colorado
3. What Is the Average Cna Salary by State. ZipRecruiter. Accessed 8 October 2024. https://www.ziprecruiter.com/Salaries/What-Is-the-Average-CNA-Salary-by-State

7. FROM HEALERS TO HUSTLERS

1. Cline, M. Defensive Medicine and the Fear of Being Sued by Patients. MedMalFirm. 14 Sept 2021. Accessed 8 October 2024. https://www.medmalfirm.com/news-and-updates/malpractice-lawsuit-fear-extra-tests/
2. Prodromos C, Rumschlag T. Hydroxychloroquine is effective, and consistently so when provided early, for COVID-19: a systematic review. New Microbes New Infect [Internet]. 2020 Oct 5 [cited 2025 May 29];38:100776. Available from: https://www.ncbi.nlm.nih.gov/pmc/articles/PMC7534595/; Neil M, Fenton N. Bayesian hypothesis testing and hierarchical modelling of ivermectin effectiveness in treating Covid-19 [Internet]. arXiv; 2021 [cited 2025 May 29]. Available from: http://arxiv.org/abs/2109.13739
3. How has U.S. spending on healthcare changed over time? [Internet]. Peterson-KFF Health System Tracker. [cited 2025 May 22]. Available from: https://www.healthsystemtracker.org/chart-collection/u-s-spending-healthcare-changed-time/

9. PREDATORY POWER

1. AHIP. New Study: In the Midst of COVID-19 Crisis, 7 out of 10 Big Pharma.... AHIP. Published October 27, 2021. https://www.ahip.org/news/articles/new-study-in-the-midst-of-covid-19-crisis-7-out-of-10-big-pharma-companies-spent-more-on-sales-and-marketing-than-r-d
2. Austin S. The Fascinating and Controversial History of Pharmaceutical Marketing. Marketing Scoop. Published May 13, 2024. Accessed October 27, 2024. https://www.marketingscoop.com/marketing/the-fascinating-and-controversial-history-of-pharmaceutical-marketing/#google_vignette
3. McGrath L. The History and Impacts of Big Pharma. The Side Unseen.

Accessed August 2, 2024. https://commons.princeton.edu/invisible-violence/the-history-and-impacts-of-big-pharma/
4. Van Zee A. The Promotion and Marketing of OxyContin: Commercial Triumph, Public Health Tragedy. Am J Public Health [Internet]. 2009 Feb [cited 2025 May 22];99(2):221–7. Available from: https://www.ncbi.nlm.nih.gov/pmc/articles/PMC2622774/
5. Direct-To-Consumer Advertising of Prescription Drugs.; 2009. Accessed October 27, 2024. https://crsreports.congress.gov/product/pdf/R/R40590
6. Affairs (ASPA) AS for P. New HHS Reports Illustrate Potential Positive Impact of Inflation Reduction Act on Prescription Drug Prices. HHS.gov. Published September 30, 2022. https://www.hhs.gov/about/news/2022/09/30/new-hhs-reports-illustrate-potential-positive-impact-inflation-reduction-act-prescription-drug-prices.html
7. Drug Prices Team. *Arnold Ventures*. 2020 [cited 2025 May 30]. "Evergreening" Stunts Competition, Costs Consumers.... Available from: https://www.arnoldventures.org/stories/evergreening-stunts-competition-costs-consumers-and-taxpayers
8. Ibid.
9. Dachs R, Darby-Stewart A, Graber M. Choosing One PPI Treatment Over Another. American Family Physician. 2007;76(9):1273-1274. https://www.aafp.org/pubs/afp/issues/2007/1101/p1273.html
10. Topol EJ. Failing the Public Health — Rofecoxib, Merck, and the FDA. New England Journal of Medicine. 2004;351(17):1707-1709. doi:https://doi.org/10.1056/nejmp048286
11. Compton K. Vioxx Lawsuits. Drugwatch.com. Published August 23, 2012. https://www.drugwatch.com/vioxx/lawsuits/
12. Compton K. Vioxx Lawsuits. Drugwatch.com. Published August 23, 2012. https://www.drugwatch.com/vioxx/lawsuits/
13. Barth M. EXCLUSIVE: Gilbert and Chattah File First Remdesivir Wrongful Death Lawsuit in Nevada. *Nevada Globe*. Published November 26, 2022. Accessed October 28, 2024. https://thenevadaglobe.com/fl/exclusive-gilbert-and-chattah-file-first-remdesivir-wrongful-death-lawsuit-in-nevada/
14. Therapeutics and COVID-19 [Internet]. World Health Organization; 2020 Nov [cited 2025 May 30]. Available from: https://iris.who.int/bitstream/handle/10665/336729/WHO-2019-nCov-remdesivir-2020.1-eng.pdf?sequence=1
15. Beigel JH, Tomashek KM, Dodd LE, et al. Remdesivir for the Treatment of Covid-19 — Final Report. New England Journal of Medicine. 2020;383(19). doi:https://doi.org/10.1056/nejmoa2007764
16. Inserro A. Gilead Sciences Sets US Price for COVID-19 Drug at $2340 to $3120 Based on Insurance. AJMC. Published June 29, 2020. https://

www.ajmc.com/view/gilead-sciences-sets-us-price-for-covid19-drug-at-2340-to-3120-based-on-insurance
17. Duke Health. Lobbying Definitions, Exceptions, and Examples | Duke Government Relations. govrelations.duke.edu. https://govrelations.duke.edu/ethics-and-compliance/lobbying-definitions-exceptions-and-examples
18. Investopedia [Internet]. [cited 2025 May 22]. Which Industry Spends the Most on Lobbying? Available from: https://www.investopedia.com/investing/which-industry-spends-most-lobbying-antm-so/
19. worldpopulationreview.com [Internet]. [cited 2025 May 22]. Healthcare Spending by Country 2025. Available from: https://worldpopulationreview.com/country-rankings/healthcare-spending-by-country
20. Fox E. How Pharma Companies Game the System to Keep Drugs Expensive. Harvard Business Review. Published April 6, 2017. https://hbr.org/2017/04/how-pharma-companies-game-the-system-to-keep-drugs-expensive
21. FDA AT A GLANCE [Internet]. Office of the Commissioner, U.S. Federal Drug Administration; 2020 Nov [cited 2025 May 22]. Available from: https://www.fda.gov/media/143704/download
22. Jewett C. F.D.A.'s Drug Industry Fees Fuel Concerns Over Influence. The New York Times [Internet]. 2022 Sep 15 [cited 2025 May 22]; Available from: https://www.nytimes.com/2022/09/15/health/fda-drug-industry-fees.html
23. Greger M. How Not to Diet: The Groundbreaking Science of Healthy, Permanent Weight Loss. Flatiron Books; 2019; Greger M. How Not to Die: Discover the Foods Scientifically Proven to Prevent and Reverse Disease. Flatiron Books, 2015; Greger M. How Not to Age: The Scientific Approach to Getting Healthier as You Get Older. Flatiron Books; 2023.

10. A SYSTEM THAT PRETENDS TO CARE

1. Lichtenstein E. The history of health insurance: Past, present, and future. AgentSync. Published October 26, 2022. Accessed August 2, 2024. https://agentsync.io/blog/health-insurance/the-history-of-health-insurance-past-present-and-future
2. U.S. Department of Health and Human Services. Who is eligible for Medicaid? HHS.gov. Published August 4, 2017. https://www.hhs.gov/answers/medicare-and-medicaid/who-is-eligible-for-medicaid/index.html
3. Tolbert J, Orgera K, Damico A. Key facts about the uninsured population. Kaiser Family Foundation. Published 2023. https://www.kff.org/uninsured/issue-brief/key-facts-about-the-uninsured-population/
4. Allen A. Patients needing home IV nutrition fear dangerous shortages. The Washington Post [Internet]. 2023 Feb 6 [cited 2025 May 23]; Avail-

able from: https://www.washingtonpost.com/health/2023/02/06/iv-nutrition-infusions-shortage/; How to Charge $546 for Six Liters of Saltwater - *The New York Times* [Internet]. [cited 2025 May 23]. Available from: https://www.nytimes.com/2013/08/27/health/exploring-salines-secret-costs.html%206-shortage/.
5. Home of the Office of Disease Prevention and Health Promotion - health.gov. Health.gov. Published 2023. https://odphp.health.gov/
6. Armstrong PRM. How Cigna Saves Millions by Having Its Doctors Reject Claims Without Reading Them. ProPublica. Published March 25, 2023. https://www.propublica.org/article/cigna-pxdx-medical-health-insurance-rejection-claims

12. A BROKEN SYSTEM AND A NATION IN CRISIS

1. Fields, S. (2023, January 17). How the world's richest people became much richer during the pandemic. Marketplace. https://www.marketplace.org/2023/01/16/how-the-worlds-richest-people-became-much-richer-during-the-pandemic/
2. Oversight Committee Republicans Verified account. (2024, June 13). Hearing wrap up: Dr. Fauci held publicly accountable by select subcommittee - United States House Committee on Oversight and Accountability. United States House Committee on Oversight and Accountability. https://oversight.house.gov/release/hearing-wrap-up-dr-fauci-held-publicly-accountable-by-select-subcommittee/
3. PowerfulJRE. Joe Rogan Experience #2255 - Mark Zuckerberg [Internet]. YouTube; 2025 Jan 10 [cited 2025 May 23]. Available from: https://www.youtube.com/watch?v=7k1ehaEobdU
4. Department for Professional Employees, AFL-CIO [Internet]. [cited 2025 May 23]. Impact of Nurse-to-Patient Ratios: Implications of the California Nurse Staffing Mandate for Other States. Available from: https://www.dpeaflcio.org/factsheets/impact-of-nurse-to-patient-ratios-implications-of-the-california-nurse-staffing-mandate-for-other-states
5. Derecho, K. C., Cafino, R., Aquino-Cafino, S. L., Isla, A., Esencia, J. A., Lactuan, N. J., Maranda, J. a. G., & Velasco, L. C. P. (2024). Technology adoption of electronic medical records in developing economies: A systematic review on physicians' perspective. Digital Health, 10. https://doi.org/10.1177/20552076231224605
6. World Health Organization: WHO. (2019, July 16). Universal health coverage. https://www.who.int/health-topics/universal-health-coverage#tab=tab_1
7. Internation Healthcare System Profiles ENGLAND. (2020, June 5). Commonwealth Fund. Retrieved March 29, 2025, from https://www.commonwealthfund.org/international-health-policy-center/countries/england

8. United Kingdom - Individual - Taxes on personal income. (n.d.). https://taxsummaries.pwc.com/united-kingdom/individual/taxes-on-personal-income
9. How does health spending in the U.S. compare to other countries? - Peterson-KFF Health System Tracker. (2024, January 23). Peterson-KFF Health System Tracker. https://www.healthsystemtracker.org/chart-collection/health-spending-u-s-compare-countries/
10. United States - Individual - Taxes on personal income. (n.d.). https://taxsummaries.pwc.com/united-states/individual/taxes-on-personal-income
11. Himmelstein, D.U., Lawless, R.M., Thorne, D., Foohey, P., & Woolhandler, S. (2019). *Medical Bankruptcy: Still Common Despite the Affordable Care Act*. American Journal of Public Health, 109(3), 431–433.
12. Galvani, A. P., Parpia, A. S., Foster, E. M., Singer, B. H., & Fitzpatrick, M. C. (2020). Improving the prognosis of health care in the USA. The Lancet, 395(10223), 524-533. https://doi.org/10.1016/s0140-6736(19)33019-3
13. Jacobson, L. (2017, July 24). How expensive would a single-payer system be? @Politifact. https://www.politifact.com/article/2017/jul/21/how-expensive-would-single-payer-system-be/
14. Budget, C. F. a. R. F. (2025, March 27). Analysis of CBO's March 2025 Long-Term Budget Outlook-2025-03-27. Committee for a Responsible Federal Budget. https://www.crfb.org/papers/analysis-cbos-march-2025-long-term-budget-outlook#:~:text=In%20nominal%20dollars%2C%20budget%20deficits,and%20are%20projected%20to%20explode.
15. U.S. National Debt clock : real time. (n.d.). https://www.usdebtclock.org/
16. Albanese, J. (2024, October 16). Roadblock to Progress: How Medicare impedes innovation. Paragon Health Institute. https://paragoninstitute.org/medicare/roadblock-to-progress-how-medicare-impedes-health-care-innovation/
17. Nazari, A. (2024). Universal Healthcare: An In-Depth Examination and Proposed Alternatives. Deleted Journal, 10(1), 18–25. https://doi.org/10.22461/jhea.1.71643
18. Other countries with universal health care don't have Canada's long wait times. (n.d.). Fraser Institute. https://www.fraserinstitute.org/commentary/other-countries-with-universal-health-care-dont-have-canadas-long-wait-times?
19. U.S. Health Care from a Global Perspective, 2022: Accelerating Spending, Worsening Outcomes. (2023). www.commonwealthfund.org. https://doi.org/10.26099/8ejy-yc74
20. Soni, A., Wherry, L. R., & Simon, K. I. (2020). How have ACA insurance expansions affected health outcomes? Findings from the literature. Health Affairs, 39(3), 371–378. https://doi.org/10.1377/hlthaff.2019.01436

www.ingramcontent.com/pod-product-compliance
Lightning Source LLC
Chambersburg PA
CBHW052127030426
42337CB00028B/5059